# A Comprehensive Guide to Insole-Based Approaches for Diabetic Foot Complications

Muhammad Nouman • Surapong Chatpun
Editors

# A Comprehensive Guide to Insole-Based Approaches for Diabetic Foot Complications

Springer

*Editors*
Muhammad Nouman
Sirindhorn School of Prosthetics and Orthotics
Faculty of Medicine, Siriraj Hospital, Mahidol University
Bangkok, Thailand

Surapong Chatpun
Department of Biomedical Sciences & Biomedical Engineering
Faculty of Medicine, Prince of Songkla University
Songkhla, Thailand

ISBN 978-981-95-0655-2 ISBN 978-981-95-0656-9 (eBook)
https://doi.org/10.1007/978-981-95-0656-9



This Springer imprint is published by the registered company Springer Nature Singapore Pte Ltd.
The registered company address is: 152 Beach Road, #21-01/04 Gateway East, Singapore 189721, Singapore

*To all the patients living with diabetes*
*around the world—*
*Your resilience inspires innovation and*
*compassion in everything we do.*
*And to our families and mentors, whose*
*unwavering support has shaped our journey.*

# Preface

The human foot is a complex mechanical structure that bears weight and allows locomotion; it is often overlooked until complications arise. For individuals living with diabetes, the foot becomes a focal point of vulnerability. Diabetic foot complications are among the most serious and costly consequences of the disease, often leading to ulcers, infections, and in severe cases, amputation. This book emerges from a growing need to fill the gaps in many aspects related to diabetic foot, including clinical understanding, design and material consideration for insoles, gait training, footwear, and technological innovation.

The primary aim of this book is to provide a comprehensive guide for healthcare professionals, researchers, students, and those involved in foot care technology and rehabilitation. It brings together evidence-based knowledge on the pathophysiology of diabetic foot, clinical assessment methods, and current standards in prevention and treatment. Emphasis is placed on the role of therapeutic footwear, insoles, and orthotic interventions, as well as the latest developments in wearable technologies, pressure mapping, and smart sensors for foot monitoring.

Each chapter is designed to build on the previous, combining medical insight with engineering and design perspectives. This interdisciplinary approach reflects the evolving nature of diabetic foot management—one that increasingly relies on collaborative innovation between clinicians, biomedical engineers, and technology developers. Whether you are a medical practitioner seeking to improve patient outcomes, a researcher exploring new materials and sensors, or a designer aiming to develop functional and user-centered footwear, this book offers insight and guidance. We hope that the knowledge shared in these pages will contribute not only to better clinical practice and innovation but also to a better quality of life for people living with diabetes worldwide.

Bangkok, Thailand — Muhammad Nouman
Songkhla, Thailand — Surapong Chatpun

# Contents

# Contributors

**Surapong Chatpun** Department of Biomedical Sciences and Biomedical Engineering, Faculty of Medicine, Prince of Songkla University, Songkhla, Thailand

**Tulaya Dissaneewate** Department of Rehabilitation Medicine, Faculty of Medicine, Prince of Songkla University, Hat Yai, Songkhla, Thailand

**Muhammad Nouman** Sirindhorn School of Prosthetics and Orthotics, Faculty of Medicine, Siriraj Hospital, Mahidol University, Bangkok, Thailand

**Pannika Prachgosin** Department of Rehabilitation Medicine, Faculty of Medicine, Siriraj Hospital, Mahidol University, Bangkok, Thailand

**Satta Srewaradachpisal** Department of Mechanical and Mechatronics Engineering, Faculty of Engineering, Prince of Songkla University, Songkhla, Thailand

# Abbreviations

| | |
|---|---|
| DFU | Diabetic Foot Ulcer |
| DPN | Diabetic Peripheral Neuropathy |
| EVA | Ethylene-Vinyl Acetate |
| PU | Polyurethane |
| AI | Artificial Intelligence |
| IoT | Internet of Things |
| CAD/CAM | Computer-Aided Design/Computer-Aided Manufacturing |
| IWGDF | International Working Group on the Diabetic Foot |
| ABI | Ankle-Brachial Index |

# Overview of Diabetic Foot Complications

# 1

Muhammad Nouman and Surapong Chatpun

## 1.1 Overview of Diabetic Foot Complications

Diabetes mellitus is a growing global health issue, with approximately 537 million individuals affected worldwide in 2021, and this number is projected to increase significantly by 2045 [1–3]. Among its myriad complications, diabetic foot problems remain one of the most debilitating and costly. Approximately 15–25% of diabetic individuals will develop a foot ulcer during their lifetime, many of which result in infection, hospitalization, or lower-limb amputation [4–6]. Diabetic foot ulcers (DFUs) are the leading cause of nontraumatic amputations globally, contributing to high healthcare expenditure and reduced quality of life. DFUs are deep tissue lesions that are associated with ischemic, neuropathic, or combined neuro-ischemic abnormalities. These complications are a leading cause of morbidity and mortality. Apart from the physical and emotional burden on patients, the healthcare system encounters rising expenses associated with hospitalization, therapeutic procedures, and prolonged care [7–9].

The socioeconomic burden of diabetic foot complications is profound. The burden of DFU impacts both direct and indirect costs for hospitalization, treatment, special footwear, rehabilitation medicine, long-term care, unemployment, transportation, and psychotherapy. In addition to the physical and emotional effect on patients, the loss of income experienced by patients and their families is considered

M. Nouman (✉)
Sirindhorn School of Prosthetics and Orthotics, Faculty of Medicine,
Siriraj Hospital, Mahidol University, Bangkok, Thailand
e-mail: muhammad.nou@mahidol.ac.th

S. Chatpun
Department of Biomedical Sciences and Biomedical Engineering, Faculty of Medicine,
Prince of Songkla University, Songkhla, Thailand



M. Nouman, S. Chatpun (eds.), *A Comprehensive Guide to Insole-Based Approaches for Diabetic Foot Complications*,
https://doi.org/10.1007/978-981-95-0656-9_1

a major cost under the direct nonmedical and indirect cost categories. According to research, treating a single DFU can cost a lot, particularly when complications including infection and amputation occur. These complications can be avoided by prompt identification, patient education, changing lifestyle, self-care practice, and a multidisciplinary approach.

## 1.2 Overview of the Structure, Functions of the Foot, and Understanding the Gait Cycle

The foot is a complex and important structure vital for movement, balance, and weight-bearing. The foot is composed of bones, joints, ligaments, tendons, muscles, nerves, and blood vessels; its intrinsic design ensures stability and flexibility. The majority of people experience foot problems, often linked to footwear, activity levels, and other health conditions. Understanding foot anatomy and biomechanics of the foot helps address issues related to injuries, surgeries, and chronic conditions like Charcot foot.

In a normal foot, bones and joints maintain structural integrity, allowing even distribution of weight and dynamic motion. The foot can be divided into several categories, including bones, joints, muscles, blood vessels, ligaments, tendons, and nerves. There are 26 bones in a foot that can be divided into three main anatomical regions: hindfoot (talus and calcaneus), midfoot (navicular, cuboid, and three cuneiform bones), and forefoot (five metatarsals and 14 phalanges) (Fig. 1.1). A sophisticated network of muscles, ligaments, nerves, blood vessels, arteries, and tendons ensures stability and facilitates mobility throughout various daily tasks. To support the foot structure, a typical foot depends on both intrinsic and extrinsic muscles to stabilize the foot, maintain fat pad alignment under the metatarsal heads, and behave

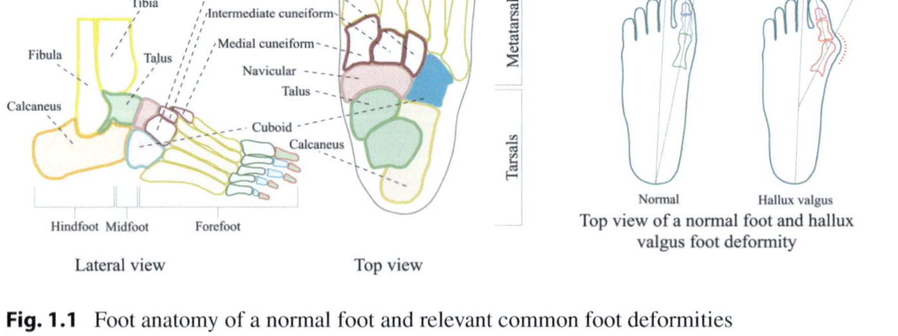


**Fig. 1.1** Foot anatomy of a normal foot and relevant common foot deformities

as a rigid structure to provide support during propulsion. In a normal foot, the ligaments and tendons remain flexible, enabling smooth joint motion. The intact sensory and motor nerves enable protective sensation, proprioception, and coordinated muscle activation throughout the gait. The micro- and macrovascular networks ensure adequate blood supply to the extremities for tissue repair and infection resistance.

On the other hand, diabetic feet exhibit various changes over time. These observations can be as severe as Charcot neuroarthropathy, a destructive process where neuropathy and repetitive trauma result in midfoot collapse, causing rocker-bottom deformity. Furthermore, chronic hyperglycemia accelerates osteopenia, reducing bone density and increasing macro- and microfracture risk. The intrinsic muscle atrophy occurs due to motor neuropathy and distal movement of fat pads and exposing metatarsal heads to elevate plantar pressure. The extrinsic muscle weakness with reduced plantar and dorsiflexion alters gait mechanics and increases reliance on compensatory gait patterns. Moreover, the stiffness of ligaments and tendons reduces flexibility, and it contributes to various toe deformities due to shortening and imbalance between flexors and extensors. In diabetic neuropathy, peripheral sensory neuropathy causes loss of protective sensation, leaving patients unaware of trauma. Motor neuropathy disrupts intrinsic and extrinsic muscle coordination, leading to toe deformities and gait instability. Autonomic neuropathy further reduces sweat gland function, causing dry, fissured skin prone to infection. In addition, peripheral disease narrows blood vessels, reducing perfusion and oxygen supply to extremities [10]. Combined with neuropathy, peripheral arterial disease creates a double-hit effect, where tissue damage progresses rapidly due to poor healing capacity (Table 1.1).

The normal human gait cycle is divided into stance (60%) and swing (40%) phases. During stance phase (initial contact to terminal stance), the foot must provide stability and forward propulsion, while swing phase requires foot clearance. Diabetic foot pathology (especially peripheral neuropathy) disrupts this. Loss of sensation and intrinsic muscle function lead to altered biomechanics; patients often demonstrate slow gait, shorter strides, and prolonged double support to compensate. The diabetic neuropathy with tibialis anterior weakness produces a steppage gait, a high-step pattern to avoid tripping due to foot drop. Intrinsic foot muscle wasting flattens the arch and reduces toe stability, further changing load distribution. These gait changes increase the risk of falls and contribute to approximately 6.6 times higher chances of developing ulceration and re-ulceration under metatarsal heads [11].

During initial contact, patients often lack heel contact due to Achilles tightness (equinus) or proprioceptive loss, resulting in an early landing of the foot instead of a normal heel strike. Loss of arch support (intrinsic muscle atrophy) leads to midfoot collapse. The tibia advances too quickly, increasing plantar pressure under metatarsal heads. Loss of protective sensation can lead to medial and lateral gait deviation. Moreover, toe deformities reduce effective toe-off during the terminal stance phase of the gait cycle. Contracted toes exert abnormally high pressure on metatarsal heads, reducing pressure redistribution and weakening propulsion. Foot

**Table 1.1** Anatomical structures and clinical relevance of normal foot and diabetic foot

| Structure | Extrinsic muscles | Intrinsic muscles | Diabetic foot |
|---|---|---|---|
| Muscle groups | ***Anterior:*** Tibialis anterior, extensor hallucis longus, extensor digitorum longus ***Posterior:*** Gastrocnemius, soleus, flexor digitorum longus, flexor hallucis longus ***Lateral:*** Fibularis longus and brevis | ***Dorsal:*** Extensor Digitorum brevis, extensor hallucis brevis ***Plantar:*** Abductor hallucis, flexor digitorum brevis, lumbricals, interossei | Atrophy of intrinsic and weak extrinsic |
| Tendons | Long tendons cross ankle: Achilles tendon, tibialis posterior tendon, peroneal tendon | Short tendons within the foot, support toe movement | Stiffness of tendons |
| Ligaments | Interact closely with: Deltoid ligament (medial), lateral ligaments, spring ligaments | Work closely with: Plantar fascia, long and short plantar ligaments | |
| Blood supply | Anterior tibial artery (dorsalis pedis), posterior tibial artery, peroneal artery | Medial and lateral arteries (branches of posterior tibial artery) | Peripheral arterial disease, ischemia, poor healing |
| Nerve supply | Deep peroneal (anterior compartment), superficial peroneal (lateral), tibial nerve (posterior) | Medial and lateral plantar nerves (from tibial nerve) | Neuropathy |
| Clinical relevance | Foot drop, Achilles tendinopathy, shin splint, important in ankle stabilization | Loss of arch support, claw toes, balance issues in neuropathy | |

drop, which results from dorsiflexion weakness, is common in diabetic foot during the swing phase. This condition leads to an inability to clear the toes, causing a compensatory steppage gait with increased flexion of hip and knee joints to avoid dragging the toes. The diabetic neuropathic patients walk with lower velocity, shorter stride length, longer stride, and stance time [12].

## 1.3 Causes, Risk Factors, and Potential Complications of Untreated Diabetic Foot

Diabetic foot complications encompass a wide range of conditions and are multifactorial, mainly due to long-term high blood glucose levels that cause damage, often involving a combination of nerve damage, poor blood flow, and infections. Peripheral neuropathy is a result of prolonged hyperglycemia that damages nerve fibers and leads to a loss of protective sensation, making individuals unaware of major or minor injuries or irregular pressure-related trauma to the foot. In parallel, peripheral arterial disease (PAD) contributes significantly to tissue ischemia as diabetes accelerates atherosclerosis, reduces blood supply to the extremities, impairs wound healing, and increases susceptibility to infections. These complications compromise skin integrity and tissue viability, leading to ulceration and potential limb loss. Neuropathic ulcers result from sensory neuropathy (loss of protective sensation), motor neuropathy (foot deformities), and autonomic neuropathy (dry skin and fissures). These ulcers commonly develop in pressure areas at the forefoot, under metatarsal heads and at the big toe due to high pressure during terminal stance.

Several factors increase the likelihood of developing diabetic foot complications. The longer duration of diabetes increases the risk of neuropathy and vascular complications. Elevated HbA1c levels or poor glycemic control also correlate with increased complication rates. Smoking exacerbates both wound healing impairment and vascular disease. Additionally, structural foot deformities, like Charcot foot and hammer toes, increase repetitive abnormal peak plantar pressure at the forefoot and midfoot regions, leading to ulceration. A previous history of ulceration significantly raises the risk of recurrence, either at the same site or in another anatomical position. These factors create a compounded effect, making individuals susceptible to serious foot issues and even amputation. If the diabetic is left untreated, it can progress to severe complications that include foot ulceration, infections, gangrene, and amputation [13, 14]. Foot calluses and ulcers are the most common clinical manifestation and can become infected, leading to deeper tissue involvement. In severe cases, poor blood flow and persistent infection can result in tissue necrosis and gangrene, ultimately necessitating partial or total amputation. These complications are directly linked with high mortality rates and reduced quality of life within 5 years of amputation.

## 1.4 Importance of Foot Care in Diabetes

Preventive foot care plays an important role in reducing the incidence and severity of diabetic foot complications. Patients should be properly educated to conduct daily foot inspection to detect early signs of redness, swelling, blisters, callus formation, or any other abnormalities. Maintaining proper hygiene through daily washing and thorough drying, especially between the toes, helps prevent fungal and bacterial infections. Applying medical grade moisturizers specific for diabetic feet can prevent skin dryness and cracking, though lotions should be avoided between the toes to reduce the risk of fungal infection and further complications.

Appropriate footwear should be properly fitted to protect the feet and avoid excessive pressure and high shear forces that are causative factor of callus formation and ulceration. Ill-fitting footwear remains one of the most frequent causes of foot ulcers in diabetic patients. It is evident that foot care education and regular screening can significantly reduce the risk of ulceration and amputation. The 5 P's framework can be indicated for better education of the patients that include prevention by regular screening and risk assessment, protection by using appropriate footwear and skincare, pressure relief by having custom-made insole to reduce and redistribute peak plantar pressure, prompt care by reporting early about or any kind of infections, and follow-ups by trained medical healthcare professional specialized in foot and ankle (Fig. 1.2). To provide the abovementioned care, the multidisciplinary team should always be encouraged including podiatrists, wound care nurses, vascular surgeons, orthotists, and prosthetists to ensure comprehensive care and improve limb salvage rates.

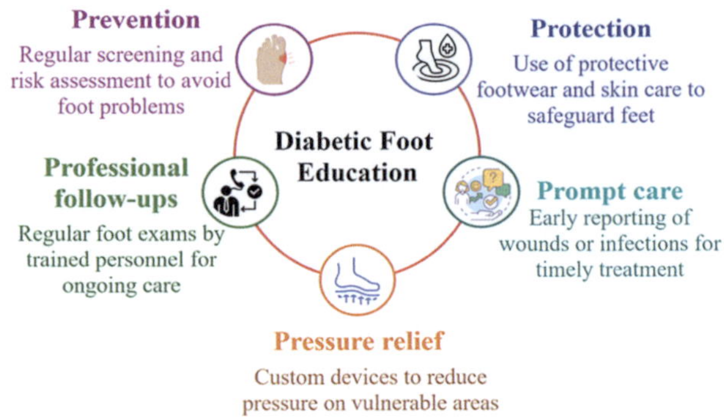


**Fig. 1.2** Foundation of diabetic foot care based on 5 P's framework

## 1.5 Clinical Assessment of Diabetic Foot Complications

Effective clinical assessment of the diabetic foot involves a structured approach that begins with a detailed history and physical examination. Clinicians should access the duration of diabetes, current glycemic control, presence of comorbidities, and any prior foot complications. Visual inspection of the foot can reveal skin changes, deformities, calluses, ulceration, or signs of infection. Palpation helps in assessing temperature differences, pulses, and capillary refill time to evaluate circulatory status.

Neurological evaluation is critical in detecting peripheral neuropathy. The 10-gram monofilament test is a commonly used tool to access the protective sensation. Additional tests include vibration perception using a tuning fork and pinprick sensation to evaluate small-fiber function. Vascular assessment includes palpating dorsalis pedis and posterior tibial pulse, calculating the ankle-brachial index (ABI), and performing Doppler ultrasound to detect arterial insufficiency. The risk factor stratification, based on clinical findings, helps guide follow-up frequency and intervention intensity. Patients without neuropathy or PAD are considered low-risk and may require annual assessments. Those with isolated neuropathy or vascular disease fall into the moderate-risk category, while individuals with previous ulcers, deformities, or prior amputation are classified as high-risk. High-risk patients require more frequent monitoring and comprehensive preventive care plans. In clinical practice, diabetic foot ulcers can be classified based on the Wagner classification, the University of Texas classification (UT), and the Wound, Ischemia, and Foot Infection (WIFi). Wagner classification is best suited for initial screening or in setting where time and resources are limited. Moreover, the University of Texas classification serves as a middle ground, combining wound depth (grade) with the presence of ischemia and infection (stage), though without the quantitative detail of WIFi. These systems overlap in evaluating wound characteristics yet differ in the depth of granularity and the independent assessment of infection and vascular compromise. These tools provide consolidated framework for clinicians to select the most appropriate classification system based on clinical context and resource availability (Table 1.2).

Additional diagnostic modalities support clinical examination in identifying at-risk feet. Thermal imaging and skin temperature monitoring can reveal inflammation before ulceration. Biothesiometry and quantitative sensory testing allow precise

**Table 1.2** Comparison of the Wagner classification, the University of Texas classification (UT), and the Wound, Ischemia, and Foot Infection (WIFi)

| Feature | Wagner | University of Texas | WIFi |
|---|---|---|---|
| Focus | Ulcer depth and extend of gangrene | Ulcer depth, presence of infection and ischemia | Comprehensive risk stratification |
| Grading | Single grade (0–5) | Combined grade (0–3) and stage (A–D) | Separate scores (0–3) for wound, ischemia, and wound infection |
| Wound assessment | Ulcer depth and gangrene and gangrene extend | Ulcer depth (grade 0–3) | Wound grade 1–3 (from superficial ulcer to extensive gangrene) |
| Ischemia | Not assessed | Presence-based (stage C or D) | Quantified via ABI or toe pressure (0 = none, 3 = severe) |
| Infection | Not accessed | Presence-based (stage B or D) | Quantify by depth/systemic signs (0 = none, 3 = systemic infection) |
| Example grade | Grade 3: Deep ulcers with abscess or osteomyelitis | Grade 2, stage D: Ulcer penetrates tendon with infection and ischemia | W1 I2 fI1: Shallow wound, moderate ischemia, mild infection |
| Grade 0 | Intact skin with bony deformity | Pre- or post-ulcerative lesion, completely epithelialized | No open wound (W0) |
| Grade 1 | Superficial ulcer | Superficial wound not involving tendon, capsule, or bone | Superficial ulcer (W1) |
| Grade 2 | Ulcer extension to tendon, bone, or joint capsule | Ulcer penetration to tendon or capsule | Deep ulcer reaching tendon/bone (W2) |
| Grade 3 | Deep ulcer with abscess or osteomyelitis | Ulcer penetration to bone or joint | Extensive ulcer, possibly gangrenous (W3) |
| Grade 4 | Partial foot gangrene | – | – |
| Grade 5 | Extensive gangrene of foot | – | – |
| Stage A | – | Clean ulcer | – |
| Stage B | – | Infected ulcer | – |
| Stage C | – | Ischemic ulcer | – |
| Stage D | – | Infected and ischemic ulcer | – |
| Clinical use | Easy to use, widely recognized | More comprehensive; considers multi-risk factors | Predicts amputation risk, guides revascularization and limb salvage strategies |
| Limitation | Does not account for infection or ischemia | More complex to use | Requires vascular assessment tools; may be too detailed for basic clinical settings |

grading of neuropathy. Toe-brachial index and transcutaneous oxygen pressure ($TcPO_2$) provide a clearer vascular picture in patient with arterial calcification. When deep infection or osteomyelitis is suspected, imaging tools like plain radiography or MRI should be employed. These investigations, combined with risk stratification systems such as IWGDF or SINBAD score, aid in tailoring preventive and therapeutic strategies to individual patients.

## References


1. Hossain MJ, Al-Mamun M, Islam MR. Diabetes mellitus, the fastest growing global public health concern: early detection should be focused. Health Sci Rep. 2024;7(3):e2004.
2. Sun H, Saeedi P, Karuranga S, Pinkepank M, Ogurtsova K, Duncan BB, et al. IDF diabetes atlas: global, regional and country-level diabetes prevalence estimates for 2021 and projections for 2045. Diabetes Res Clin Pract. 2022;183:109119.
3. Ong KL, Stafford LK, McLaughlin SA, Boyko EJ, Vollset SE, Smith AE, et al. Global, regional, and national burden of diabetes from 1990 to 2021, with projections of prevalence to 2050: a systematic analysis for the global burden of disease study 2021. Lancet. 2023;402(10397):203–34.
4. Yazdanpanah L, Nasiri M, Adarvishi S. Literature review on the management of diabetic foot ulcer. World J Diabetes. 2015;6(1):37–53.
5. Gershater MA, Löndahl M, Nyberg P, Larsson J, Thörne J, Eneroth M, et al. Complexity of factors related to outcome of neuropathic and neuroischaemic/ischaemic diabetic foot ulcers: a cohort study. Diabetologia. 2009;52(3):398–407.
6. Ikura K, Hanai K, Oka S, Watanabe M, Oda Y, Hamada M, et al. Brachial-ankle pulse wave velocity, but not ankle-brachial index, predicts all-cause mortality in patients with diabetes after lower extremity amputation. J Diabetes Investig. 2017;8(2):250–3.
7. Fejfarová V, Koliba M, Piťhová P, Flekač M, Prýmková V, Venerová J, et al. Economic burden of podiatric care for diabetic foot ulcers in The Czech Republic: a prospective multicenter study. Diabetes Res Clin Pract. 2025;223:112141.
8. Hashempour R, MirHashemi S, Mollajafari F, Damiri S, ArabAhmadi A, Raei B. Economic burden of diabetic foot ulcer: a case of Iran. BMC Health Serv Res. 2024;24(1):363.
9. Da Ros R, Assaloni R, Michelli A, Brunato B, Barro E, Meloni M, et al. Burden of infected diabetic foot ulcers on hospital admissions and costs in a third-level center. Ann Vasc Surg. 2024;5(2):141–50.
10. Differential Diagnosis of Abnormal Symptoms and Signs. In: Ettinger AB, Weisbrot DM, editors. Neurologic differential diagnosis: a case-based approach. Cambridge: Cambridge University Press; 2014. p. 1–546.
11. Lázaro-Martínez J, Aragón-Sánchez J, Alvaro-Afonso F, García-Morales E, García-Álvarez Y, Molines-Barroso R. The best way to reduce reulcerations: if you understand biomechanics of the diabetic foot, you can do it. Int J Low Extrem Wounds. 2014;13:294.
12. Wang Z, Peng S, Zhang H, Sun H, Hu J. Gait parameters and peripheral neuropathy in patients with diabetes: a meta-analysis. Front Endocrinol. 2022;13:891356.
13. Bansod H, Wanjari A, Dumbhare O. A review on relationship between Charcot Neuroarthropathy and diabetic patients. Cureus. 2023;15(12):e50988.
14. Lipsky BA, Senneville É, Abbas ZG, Aragón-Sánchez J, Diggle M, Embil JM, et al. Guidelines on the diagnosis and treatment of foot infection in persons with diabetes (IWGDF 2019 update). Diabetes Metab Res Rev. 2020;36(Suppl 1):e3280.

# Insoles for Diabetic Foot Complications 2

Muhammad Nouman and Surapong Chatpun

## 2.1 Introduction to Insoles

Diabetic foot complications, which involve neuropathy, formation of ulcers, and infection, affect millions globally. The complications can cause serious outcomes, which involve limb amputation as well as limitations in mobility. Peripheral neuropathy is common in diabetic patients, which lowers foot sensation, making them more likely to be injured as well as develop foot ulcers [1–3]. Furthermore, diabetic patients' poor blood supply can hinder healing from wounds, making infections as well as amputations more likely to be seen in severe cases. Diabetic foot ulceration becomes a leading cause of nontraumatic lower limb amputation [3–5]. To mitigate these risks, it is crucial for diabetic individuals to regularly check their feet for any signs of injury or infection. Implementing a comprehensive foot care routine, along with custom insoles, can greatly enhance mobility and overall quality of life (Fig. 2.1). Insoles, also referred to as foot orthoses, are inserts that are placed in shoes in order to give additional support and cushioning, as well as redistributions of plantar pressure. In diabetic foot care, insoles are essential in preventing ulcers as well as other foot complications.

Principles of torque, pressure, and force translate directly into insole design as well as functionality. The success of foot orthoses is dependent on their functionality in distributing efficient plantar pressure. Customized insoles can be utilized in

M. Nouman (✉)
Sirindhorn School of Prosthetics and Orthotics, Faculty of Medicine,
Siriraj Hospital, Mahidol University, Bangkok, Thailand
e-mail: muhammad.nou@mahidol.ac.th

S. Chatpun
Department of Biomedical Sciences and Biomedical Engineering, Faculty of Medicine,
Prince of Songkla University, Songkhla, Thailand



M. Nouman, S. Chatpun (eds.), *A Comprehensive Guide to Insole-Based Approaches for Diabetic Foot Complications*,
https://doi.org/10.1007/978-981-95-0656-9_2

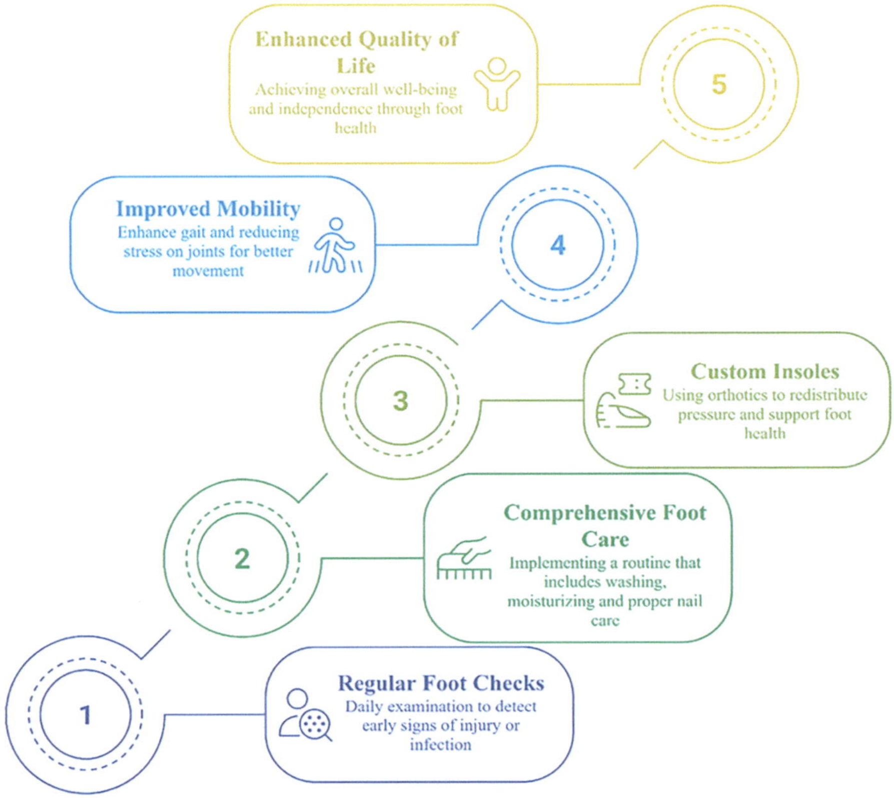


**Fig. 2.1** Steps to prevent diabetic foot complications

order to minimize peak plantar pressure by maximizing contact area [6, 7]. But that kind of relief from pressure cannot totally counteract the underlying biomechanical foot dysfunction impacts on plantar pressure distribution as well as on mechanical tissue stress. Moving the center of pressure around during walking can make diabetic foot problems worse. This puts more stress on certain areas like the metatarsal heads. Foot orthosis (FO) is very important for diabetic foot care because of redistribution of plantar pressure. FO keeps sensitive areas of the foot from getting too much abnormal peak pressure. Furthermore, FO aids in aligning foot posture, accommodating deforming areas, as well as providing a form of mechanical assistance in order to limit excessive joint motion. Pressure redistribution is critical in preventing ulcers from forming, which is a prime cause of diabetic foot hospitalizations as well as amputation. FO aids in improving gait mechanics as well as in shearing forces' diminishment, which can also contribute toward ulcers [8]. Clinically and biomechanically, FO are designed to address the specific needs of diabetic patients by providing cushioning, accomodating foot deformities, and relieving pressure. FO application is often a component in a complete diabetic foot care strategy that includes regular foot examination, suitable footwear, and patient education.

## 2.2 Classification of Foot Orthoses

The purpose of FO is to promote comfort, provide support, and treat biomechanical foot deformities. We generally divide FO into accommodating FO and functional FO, subclassifying them according to customization level according to requirements. Accommodating FO generally provides cushioning as well as relief to fixed deformities, whereas functional FO is made with a design that aims to correct foot posture as well as overall foot functioning. Knowing about these categories can assist in selecting a suitable FO according to an individual requirement in terms of function, material, and offloading technique. The division is made on a basis that insoles cater to a broad category of foot structures; prefabricated insoles are mass-produced, giving comfort as well as slight functionality in order to minimize as well as rectify overall foot posture. But specially made insoles treat a broad category of foot complexities. In case a person is involved in a job that demands standing as well as repeated activities, insoles with additional cushioning as well as a supportive arch give a more effective distribution of plantar load [9]. Insoles are also categorized based on the severity of deformities. The design of accommodating insoles primarily focuses on providing comfort, distributing load, and enhancing cushioning. Such insoles are specifically suitable in case a person suffers from diabetes as well as in case a patient presents high-plantar areas with a static deformity. The insoles distribute load, which relieves high areas from load as well as decreases ulcers as well as calluses formation. The insoles are made from soft material that comprises memory foam, ethylene vinyl acetate (EVA), as well as gel [10, 11]. Such insoles give excellent cushioning as well as comfort. Furthermore, they also prevent foot complications in diabetic or neuropathy patients, making functional insoles a necessary consideration in those suffering from chronic foot conditions. Specifically designed to manage abnormal foot motion, functional insoles improve both gait and foot positioning. Functional insoles assist in positioning the foot correctly in order to enhance balance as well as minimize strain, making functional insoles a beneficial fit for those suffering from foot conditions such as flexible foot deformities. Functional insoles prevent excessive turning inward or outward of the foot by stabilizing the arch as well as aligning the heel. This halts pain as well as minimizes common foot issues such as Achilles tendonitis and shin splints. Functional insoles also aid in maintaining overall joint health by improving walking patterns, which minimizes the possibility of injury in knees as well as hips. Therefore, users are likely to enjoy increased comfort in daily activities as well as enhanced sporting performances. Depending on classification, material selection is critical in terms of shock absorption, pressure distribution, and realignment functionality, as well as durability. Custom insoles generally employ a vast array of materials. Such material ranges from EVA, which is highly cushioning as well as light in weight, to polyurethane, which is extremely durable as well as firm in its support. Furthermore, silicone gel material is highly effective in shock absorption as well as in relief from pressure. In contrast, stiff EVA with a high shore value, along with other material combinations, offer both cushioning and stability as well as enhanced durability [12, 13]. Apart from these materials, some customized insoles also employ advanced technologies in terms of moisture-wicking material as well as antimicrobial treatments in order to boost comfort as well as hygiene [14]. By having insole composition tailored to an individual requirement, users are able to greatly enhance overall foot health as well as reduce risks of injury. Not only does a tailored approach allow for enhanced alignment, but it also enhances activity performance. As a consequence, users are able to have more comfort in daily activities, leading to a quality life. Life is also made more enjoyable with the prospect of customized foot solutions that are tailored to a person's foot shape as well as condition. Such a level of customization allows an individual foot shape pain-free experience, which encourages users toward more physical activity as well as participation in daily activities. Making physical activity more accessible also fosters a sense of belonging and peer encouragement. In the end, a tailored approach not only ensures physical health but also overall happiness.

## 2.3 Mechanisms of Action of Insoles in Offloading Peak Plantar Pressure

One of the critical functions served by insoles is redistributing peak plantar pressure over foot surface in a manner that does not lead to excessive load on areas. The conformity with foot shape by soft material distributes load over equal areas, removing localized load on high-risk areas, especially on the forefoot. Not just improving comfort, it also reduces risks of acquiring foot condition such as plantar fasciitis or metatarsalgia [15–17]. Apart from cushioning, insoles can also greatly contribute toward overall foot health as well as overall mobility. Custom insoles consider foot biomechanics in each foot, which allows compensation in a tailored manner in order to reduce peak plantar pressure. Not just enhancing comfort, a tailored approach also ensures enhanced positioning as well as functioning in motion. In correcting specified requirements, insoles can greatly contribute to overall foot health as well as reduce the risk of injury. In varying insole shape, material density, and insole thickness, as well as in shaping arches, insoles made specifically are tailored in order to achieve optimized pressure offloading according to each wearer. Studies have confirmed that insoles with metatarsal pads reduce peak plantar pressure in high-risk areas by as much as 33.1% [18, 19]. In addition, impact loads developed in walking as well as in running can cause joint aching as well as musculoskeletal load. To counteract these impacts, insoles made specifically can absorb as well as distribute these loads more evenly over the foot, hence enhancing comfort as well as improving biomechanics. Therefore, users tend toward enhanced performances in activities as well as a great alleviation of aching over time.

Insoles made from shock-absorbing material counteract these loads by cushioning the foot. Studies have confirmed that polyurethane insoles reduce impact load on joints by 22.4% in comparison with common foam insoles [20, 21]. When walking on a horizontal surface, a combination of varying material densities lowered peak plantar pressure in toes as well as forefoot by 26% and 24%, respectively [22, 23]. Custom insoles do this by widening the midfoot contact area, which distributes loads as well as lowers high-risk area pressures. Not only does this innovative approach enhance comfort, but it also lowers the risk of acquiring common foot conditions plantar fasciitis as well as metatarsalgia. Due to these developments, athletes, as well as those with demanding lifestyles, are increasingly looking toward these advanced insoles in order to boost performance as well as overall foot condition. Targeting specific biomechanics, these insoles are able to greatly enhance sporting performance as well as guard against injury. Furthermore, extended benefits from wearing customized insoles are observed far into the distant future, as improved foot positioning as well as stability are attained with regular activities. This can translate into increased stamina as well as a lack of tiredness, which means that users are able to train longer as well as more efficiently. Because awareness is on the increase regarding these benefits, more are looking toward investing in quality foot care in both daily activities and sporting activities.

## 2.4 Clinical Assessment, Evaluation, and Prescription of Insoles

The prescription of insoles involves a thorough clinical assessment, which includes patient history, gait analysis, plantar pressure mapping, and foot structure examination. Healthcare professionals, podiatrists, and orthopedic specialists access plantar pressure distribution using pedobarographic and in-shoe pressure measurement systems. A scientific approach includes understanding lower limb biomechanics, identifying areas of excessive plantar pressure, determining the desired function of the insole, and using appropriate impression techniques and insole materials. The prescription of insoles depends on factors such as foot deformity, level of mobility, and pressure distribution abnormalities [24, 25]. Conditions requiring specific corrections prescribe custom-made insoles, while general foot support and mild pressure relief recommend prefabricated insoles. To design an effective insole, certain key considerations should include an understanding and evaluation of the biomechanics of the lower limb, identification of excessive pressure areas, determination of the desired function of the insole, utilization of appropriate impression techniques, and selection of appropriate insole materials.

## 2.5 Evidence for the Effectiveness of Insoles in Managing Diabetic Foot Complications

Insoles are essential for the management of diabetic foot complications, as they reduce plantar pressure, prevent the formation of ulcers, and improve foot function. According to research, in-shoe plantar pressure analysis can improve and maintain the offloading capacity of custom-made footwear for high-risk patients [6]. This lowers the risk of diabetic foot ulcers caused by pressure reduction. Both custom-made and prefabricated orthotics have been demonstrated to be effective in reducing the risk of ulcers in individuals with diabetes and neuropathy. Prefabricated insoles are a more cost-effective solution with similar peak pressure reduction capabilities, unlike custom-made insoles, which provide tailored support and pressure redistribution. The effectiveness of custom-made insoles in substantially reducing peak pressures and force-time integrals in the heel and first metatarsal head regions has been demonstrated. Simultaneously, they elevate pressures and integrals in the medial midfoot region, thereby redistributing burdens to more secure regions of the foot. The efficacy of these insoles is further improved by plantar pressure measurements, which offer essential data for the development of insoles that optimize peak pressure reduction. In patients with neuropathy who are at a high risk of foot ulceration, customized total contact orthoses (TCO) have been demonstrated to be highly effective in reducing peak plantar pressure during a variety of walking activities. Another critical aspect of insole design is the efficacy of offloading. Research indicates that the offloading capacity of both CAD-CAM-designed and handmade insoles is substantially enhanced by data-driven modifications. Virtual optimization has emerged as a promising technique in the insole design process as a result of technological advancements. Researchers have demonstrated that this method enhances offloading performance compared to conventional, shape-based devices, with virtually optimized orthotics exhibiting significant reductions in peak pressures [26, 27]. The insole top cover's material and fabrication are also critical factors in pressure relief. Research suggests that the maximal pressures experienced during walking are directly influenced by the thickness of the insole top cover. Although six-millimeter-thick foams provide greater pressure relief than three-millimeter-thick foams, the selection of insole top cover materials is frequently determined by factors such as availability, durability, cost-effectiveness, hygiene properties, and convenience of use, rather than solely pressure relief capacity [28]. Therapeutic footwear has been demonstrated to decrease the incidence of new ulceration and lower amputation rates in individuals with diabetes, in addition to the insoles themselves. The incorporation of viscoelastic orthotics offers supplementary advantages by substantially decreasing the mean peak pressure. Research suggests that therapeutic insoles are an essential component of diabetic foot care, as they can reduce plantar pressures by an additional 5.4–20.1% at ulcer sites in comparison to prefabricated insoles [29, 30].

## 2.6 Benefits of Using Insoles for Diabetic Foot Complications

The advantages of insoles for diabetic foot complications encompass more than just pressure relief. Insoles facilitate the even distribution of plantar pressure, thereby minimizing localized stress on regions prone to ulceration [31]. Significant shock absorption is provided by materials such as EVA and polyurethane, which mitigate impact forces and prevent excessive strain on foot tissues [32]. Insoles enhance gait and stability by providing structural support, which improves balance and decreases the risk of falls, especially in diabetic patients with neuropathy [33].

The prevention of ulcers is a significant benefit of insoles. Insoles mitigate peak pressure in critical areas of the foot, thereby preventing the development of diabetic foot ulcers, a primary contributor to lower limb amputations in diabetic patients [34]. Custom insoles offer personalized support, promoting optimal comfort and alleviating pressure for individuals with significant foot deformities [28]. This customization is especially advantageous for patients with Charcot feet, severe arch collapses, or notable foot abnormalities necessitating specialized interventions.

Insoles for diabetic foot complications are designed to alleviate pressure points, reduce friction, and prevent ulcers in vulnerable areas of the foot as well as improving mobility. Custom insoles can help stabilize foot posture, reduce friction, and mitigate the impact of neuropathy-related gait abnormalities. Insoles made from cushioned materials such as EVA foam or gel can absorb impact forces during walking, reducing the risk of tissue damage, and providing comfort for neuropathic feet. Custom insoles as well as prefabricated insoles have both worked effectively, with high-risk patients faring much better with custom insoles.

## References

1. Khumchum N, Koonalinthip N, Janchai S. Accuracy and reliability of the Ipswich touch test in identifying loss of protective sensation among diabetic patients. Foot. 2024;61:102132.
2. McLaren A-M, Lu SH. Interprofessional validation of the ipswich touch test in adults with diabetes: the Canadian experience. Can J Diabetes. 2023;47(1):38–42.
3. McDermott K, Fang M, Boulton AJM, Selvin E, Hicks CW. Etiology, epidemiology, and disparities in the burden of diabetic foot ulcers. Diabetes Care. 2022;46(1):209–21.
4. Rodrigues BT, Vangaveti VN, Urkude R, Biros E, Malabu UH. Prevalence and risk factors of lower limb amputations in patients with diabetic foot ulcers: a systematic review and meta-analysis. Diabetes Metab Syndr Clin Res Rev. 2022;16(2):102397.
5. Chamberlain RC, Fleetwood K, Wild SH, Colhoun HM, Lindsay RS, Petrie JR, et al. Foot ulcer and risk of lower limb amputation or death in people with diabetes: a national population-based retrospective cohort study. Diabetes Care. 2021;45(1):83–91.
6. Nouman M, Dissaneewate T, Leelasamran W, Chatpun S. The insole materials influence the plantar pressure distributions in diabetic foot with neuropathy during different walking activities. Gait Posture. 2019;74:154–61.
7. Nouman M, Leelasamran W, Chatpun S. Effectiveness of total contact orthosis for plantar pressure redistribution in neuropathic diabetic patients during different walking activities. Foot Ankle Int. 2017;38(8):901–8.
8. Lavery LA, LaFontaine J, Higgins KR, Lanctot DR, Constantinides G. Shear-reducing insoles to prevent foot ulceration in high-risk diabetic patients. Adv Skin Wound Care. 2012;25(11):519.
9. Anderson J, Williams AE, Nester C. Development and evaluation of a dual density insole for people standing for long periods of time at work. J Foot Ankle Res. 2020;13(1):42.
10. Shi QQ, Li PL, Yick K-L, Li N-W, Jiao J. Effects of contoured insoles with different materials on plantar pressure offloading in diabetic elderly during gait. Sci Rep. 2022;12(1):15395.
11. Collings R, Freeman J, Latour JM, Paton J. Footwear and insole design features for offloading the diabetic at risk foot – a systematic review and meta-analyses. Endocrinol Diabetes Metab. 2021;4(1):e00132.
12. Shimazaki Y, Nozu S, Inoue T. Shock-absorption properties of functionally graded EVA laminates for footwear design. Polym Test. 2016;54:98.

13. Anggoro PW, Bawono B, Jamari J, Tauviqirrahman M, Bayuseno A. Advanced design and manufacturing of custom orthotics insoles based on hybrid Taguchi-response surface method. Heliyon. 2021;7:e06481.
14. Dejene BK, Abtew MA, Birlie AA, Woldeab ME. Three-dimensional (3D) knitted spacer textile materials for advanced healthcare solutions: a comprehensive review. J Ind Text. 2024;54:15280837241290169.
15. Mendes AAMT, Silva HJA, Costa ARA, Pinheiro YT, Lins CAA, de Souza MC. Main types of insoles described in the literature and their applicability for musculoskeletal disorders of the lower limbs: a systematic review of clinical studies. J Bodyw Mov Ther. 2020;24(4):29–36.
16. Bartolo D, Galea AM, Formosa C, Gatt A. The management of metatarsalgia in rheumatoid arthritis using simple insoles: an effective concurrent treatment to drug therapy. J Am Podiatr Med Assoc. 2022;112(3):18–002.
17. Zhao X, Wang M, Fekete G, Baker JS, Wiltshire H, Gu Y. Analyzing the effect of an arch support functional insole on walking and jogging in young, healthy females. Technol Health Care. 2021;29(6):1141–51.
18. Hellstrand Tang U, Zügner R, Lisovskaja V, Karlsson J, Hagberg K, Tranberg R. Comparison of plantar pressure in three types of insole given to patients with diabetes at risk of developing foot ulcers – a two-year, randomized trial. J Clin Transl Endocrinol. 2014;1(4):121–32.
19. Brodtkorb T-H, Kogler GF, Arndt A. The influence of metatarsal support height and longitudinal axis position on plantar foot loading. Clin Biomech. 2008;23(5):640–7.
20. Jia R, Wang F, Jiang J, Zhang H, Li J. The biomechanical effects of insoles with different cushioning on the knee joints of people with different body mass index grades. Front Bioeng Biotechnol. 2023;11:1241171.
21. Melia G, Siegkas P, Levick J, Apps C. Insoles of uniform softer material reduced plantar pressure compared to dual-material insoles during regular and loaded gait. Appl Ergon. 2021;91:103298.
22. Haris F, Liau B-Y, Jan Y-K, Akbari VBH, Primanda Y, Lin K-H, et al. A review of the plantar pressure distribution effects from insole materials and at different walking speeds. Appl Sci. 2021;11(24):11851.
23. Mueller MJ, Hastings M, Commean PK, Smith KE, Pilgram TK, Robertson D, et al. Forefoot structural predictors of plantar pressures during walking in people with diabetes and peripheral neuropathy. J Biomech. 2003;36(7):1009–17.
24. Bednarczyk E, Sikora S, Kossobudzka-Górska A, Jankowski K, Hernandez-Rodriguez Y. Understanding flat feet: An in-depth analysis of orthotic solutions. J Orthop Rep. 2024;3(1):100250.
25. Bus SA. Foot structure and footwear prescription in diabetes mellitus. Diabetes Metab Res Rev. 2008;24(S1):S90–S5.
26. Telfer S, Woodburn J, Collier A, Cavanagh P. Virtually optimized insoles for offloading the diabetic foot: a randomized crossover study. J Biomech. 2017;60:157.
27. D'Amico M, Kinel E, Roncoletta P, Gnaldi A, Ceppitelli C, Belli F, et al. Data-driven CAD-CAM vs traditional total contact custom insoles: a novel quantitative-statistical framework for the evaluation of insoles offloading performance in diabetic foot. PLoS One. 2021;16(3):e0247915.
28. Bus SA, Busch-Westbroek TE, Pulles J, van Dun T, Szabo G, Lacorte DH, et al. Pressure-relieving effect of different insole top covers in people with diabetes at high risk of foot ulceration. Sensors (Basel, Switzerland). 2024;24(17):5549.
29. Mondal S, Lodh M, Sahoo S, Paul K, Biswas D, Krishna C, et al. Prevalence and predictors of infected diabetic foot ulcers (DFU) and DFU-related osteomyelitis amongst industrial workers wearing occupational safety footwear. Sci Rep. 2025;15(1):2576.
30. Ahmed S, Barwick A, Butterworth P, Nancarrow S. Footwear and insole design features that reduce neuropathic plantar forefoot ulcer risk in people with diabetes: a systematic literature review. J Foot Ankle Res. 2020;13(1):30.
31. Mueller MJ. Application of plantar pressure assessment in footwear and insert design. J Orthop Sports Phys Ther. 1999;29(12):747–55.

32. Hong WH, Lee YH, Lin YH, Tang SF, Chen HC. Effect of shoe heel height and total-contact insert on muscle loading and foot stability while walking. Foot Ankle Int. 2013;34(2):273–81.
33. Hessert MJ, Vyas M, Leach J, Hu K, Lipsitz LA, Novak V. Foot pressure distribution during walking in young and old adults. BMC Geriatr. 2005;5(1):8.
34. Boulton AJM. Pressure and the diabetic foot: clinical science and offloading techniques. Am J Surg. 2004;187(5, Supplement 1):S17–24.

# Design and Material Considerations for Insoles

# 3

Satta Srewaradachpisal, Muhammad Nouman, and Surapong Chatpun

## 3.1 Understanding Insole Design

Insole is the part inside the shoe that is in contact between the sole of the foot and the shoe. Most shoe manufacturers design it so that it can be removed and replaced. Insole design plays a crucial role in providing comfort, support, and addressing specific foot conditions. Understanding the principles behind insole design can help in selecting or creating insoles tailored to individual needs. From now on, there is still the development and design of insoles to have special capabilities in use to meet the needs of some user groups, especially the health group. When separated by production, insoles can be divided into two main groups: custom-made and pre-made insoles.

Custom-made insoles are ideal for individuals with specific or severe foot conditions, requiring precise support and a tailored fit (Fig. 3.1). They offer higher personalization and medical supervision but come at a higher cost and require more time. Pre-made insoles are suitable for general use and those with less specific needs or foot issues. They are more affordable and readily available but may not provide the same level of support or durability as custom options. Ultimately, the choice between custom-made and pre-made insoles depends on the individual's foot health

S. Srewaradachpisal
Department of Mechanical and Mechatronics Engineering, Faculty of Engineering, Prince of Songkla University, Songkhla, Thailand
e-mail: satta.s@psu.ac.th

M. Nouman
Sirindhorn School of Prosthetics and Orthotics, Faculty of Medicine, Siriraj Hospital, Mahidol University, Bangkok, Thailand

S. Chatpun (✉)
Department of Biomedical Sciences and Biomedical Engineering, Faculty of Medicine, Prince of Songkla University, Songkhla, Thailand
e-mail: surapong.c@psu.ac.th





M. Nouman, S. Chatpun (eds.), *A Comprehensive Guide to Insole-Based Approaches for Diabetic Foot Complications*,
https://doi.org/10.1007/978-981-95-0656-9_3

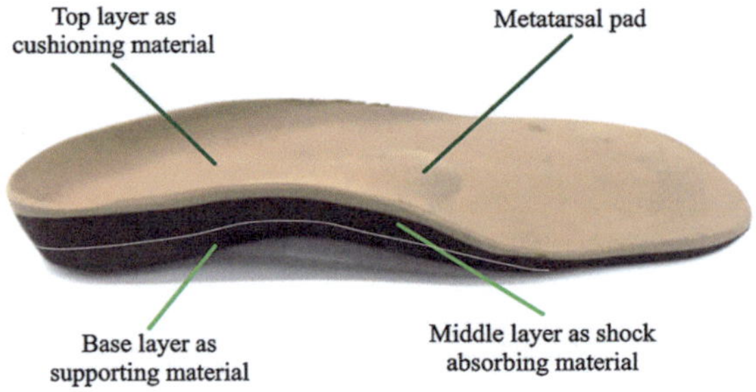


**Fig. 3.1** Custom-made insole components and design

needs, budget, and preference for convenience versus precision. For serious or chronic foot issues, consulting a healthcare professional to explore custom-made options may be the best course of action.

## 3.2 The Component of Insoles

Top cover (upper layer) of the insole is the top part of the insole that directly contacts the sole of the wearer's foot [1]. The main functions of the top cover are as follows: comfort, increases comfort for the sole and reduces impact and friction; ventilation, helps drain moisture and sweat to prevent odor and fungus; and support, helps distribute weight and pressure evenly, reducing fatigue and pain [2]. Cushioning layer of the insole is the layer between the top cover and the base of the insole. The main functions of the cushioning layer are as follows: shock absorption, helps reduce the impact that occurs while walking or running, making it feel soft and comfortable and reducing the risk of injury; weight distribution, helps distribute the weight of the body evenly, reducing pressure on any point of the sole of the foot; and support, helps support the shape of the sole of the foot and increase stability while walking or running [3, 4].

Support layer (arch and heel support) of the insole is a layer designed to support the arch of the foot (arch) and the heel (heel) specifically. Heel cup is a part designed to support and protect the heel specifically. The main functions of the heel cup are as follows: heel support, helps support and distribute weight on the heel, reducing pressure and risk of injury; stability, helps increase stability when walking or running, reducing the chance of injury from incorrect movement; and anti-slip, helps prevent the heel from slipping inside the shoe, increasing stability in movement [2, 5]. Arch support helps support the arch of the foot. Reduce the risk of arch pain and problems related to walking or running [2, 6, 7]. Metatarsal pad of the insole is a small pad designed to relieve pain and discomfort in the front of the foot, specifically. The main function of the metatarsal pad is pressure distribution. It helps distribute pressure on the metatarsal bones, reducing the risk of pain and inflammation [8]. Arch support and elevation help to lift and support the arch of the foot, making walking or running more comfortable. It also helps relieve pain from conditions such as metatarsalgia and neuromas [9]. Toe box of the insole is the part that covers the front of the shoe, which matches the area where our toes are. The main functions of the toe box are to protect the toes from impact and friction, reducing the risk of injury. The toe box provides more space for the toes, providing comfort and reducing constriction. The ventilation helps wick away moisture, preventing odor and fungus.

Bottom layer (outsole) of the insole is the lowest layer that directly contacts the inner sole (midsole). The main functions of the bottom layer are as follows: durability enhancement, helps increase the durability of the insole, making it usable for longer; grip, helps the insole grip the sole well, preventing it from slipping during use; and shock absorption, helps enhance the shock absorption from the cushioning layer, making walking or running smoother.

## 3.3 The Customer to User Insoles

The first group includes individuals who seek insoles to enhance comfort, improve performance, and reduce the risk of injuries. Athletes require highly flexible and shock-absorbing insoles to minimize impact forces and prevent injuries during high-impact activities. Older adults benefit from stable insoles designed to improve balance and reduce the risk of falls. Individuals with arthritis need insoles that evenly distribute pressure across the foot to alleviate joint pain and discomfort. People with neurological disorders require specialized insoles that assist with balance and gait stability. Individuals with gait abnormalities rely on corrective insoles to improve movement efficiency and reduce strain on the musculoskeletal system. These users may not have preexisting foot conditions but seek insoles to enhance overall comfort, mobility, and quality of life.

The second group comprises individuals with medical conditions requiring specialized insoles for foot protection, pain relief, or biomechanical correction. Key subgroups include diabetic patients, who require specialized insoles that help prevent foot ulcers by distributing pressure evenly and reducing localized stress on sensitive areas, and individuals with foot deformities, such as flat feet, high arches, and plantar fasciitis, who benefit from custom-designed insoles that provide adequate arch support and effective pressure redistribution [1, 10].

## 3.4 Design of Insole Shape

This section will discuss the results of insole shape design, which affects the human feet and body as follows. In the insole plan, there can be many shapes combined to provide functions that cover the needs of the user. Here is a classification of the foot problems. The type foot problems require customized support to improve comfort, alleviate pain, or address gait abnormalities. The special shapes of the insole parts are shown in Table 3.1.

Patients may present with a combination of illnesses that predispose them to foot issues, particularly in individuals with diabetes, whose condition induces foot weakness, hence increasing the likelihood of severe symptoms and a heightened risk of amputation.

**Table 3.1** Function of insole shape

| |
|---|
| *Arch support*<br>Arch support is essential for maintaining proper foot alignment, reducing strain on the plantar fascia, and promoting overall stability. Different levels of arch support cater to varying foot types and biomechanical needs:<br>*High arch support*<br>Designed for individuals with high arches<br>Promotes even weight distribution and reduces pressure on the heel and forefoot<br>Prevents supination (outward rolling) and enhances stability<br>*Low arch/flat support*<br>Provides adequate support for flat feet or low arches<br>Prevents overpronation (inward rolling), reducing stress on the ankles, knees, and hips<br>Arch support is particularly beneficial for improving balance and reducing pain in older adults. By providing proper foot alignment, it helps in stabilizing movements, minimizing discomfort, and preventing falls. A well-designed arch support system ensures that weight is distributed evenly, decreasing the risk of foot fatigue and musculoskeletal stress. |
| *Heel cup shape*<br>The shape and depth of the heel cup play a crucial role in foot stabilization, impact absorption, and overall comfort. Heel cup design affects how forces are transmitted through the foot during weight-bearing activities, influencing gait mechanics and reducing strain on the lower extremities.<br>*Deep heel cup*<br>Cradles the heel, stabilizing the foot and enhancing alignment<br>Reduces heel pressure and absorbs shock, which is beneficial for individuals with plantar fasciitis or heel spurs<br>Helps in controlling excessive heel movement, reducing the risk of overpronation or supination<br>*Shallow heel cup*<br>Provides more flexibility but less stability, suitable for individuals who do not require significant support<br>Allows greater freedom of motion, making it ideal for casual footwear or activities that demand increased foot mobility<br>A well-structured heel cup contributes to enhanced biomechanical efficiency by ensuring proper weight distribution and reducing localized pressure points on the heel. It plays a key role in minimizing stress transmission through the musculoskeletal system, ultimately aiding in injury prevention and improved walking mechanics. |

(continued)

**Table 3.1** (continued)

| |
|---|
| *Forefoot shape*<br>The forefoot shape of an insole affects toe splay, pressure distribution, and overall comfort. A properly designed forefoot section can alleviate pain, improve weight distribution, and enhance stability. Two common design variations include:<br>*Metatarsal pad or lift*<br>Built-in padding under the ball of the foot relieves pressure and discomfort.<br>Useful for conditions like metatarsalgia or Morton's neuroma.<br>*Flat forefoot*<br>Distributes pressure evenly across the toes and forefoot<br>Suitable for individuals who need a neutral footbed without localized pressure points<br>A well-designed forefoot section ensures proper weight transfer during gait, reducing strain on the metatarsals and preventing discomfort from prolonged standing or high-impact activities. |
| *Length of the insole*<br>The insole length determines the level of coverage and support provided to the foot. Selecting the appropriate length depends on the type of footwear and the user's specific needs:<br>*Full-length insoles*<br>Extend from the heel to the toes, offering comprehensive support<br>Ideal for closed shoes and high-impact activities<br>*3/4-length insoles*<br>Focus on the heel and arch, leaving the toes free<br>Suitable for shoes with less space, like dress shoes<br>Full-length insoles provide maximum cushioning and support for the entire foot, making them suitable for sports shoes, work boots, and orthopedic applications. Meanwhile, 3/4-length insoles offer flexibility and compatibility with tighter-fitting footwear, ensuring arch and heel support without crowding the toe box. |
| *Contour and curvature*<br>The contour and curvature of an insole significantly influence comfort, support, and biomechanical correction. Different levels of contouring provide varying benefits:<br>*Highly contoured insoles*<br>Designed to match the natural curves of the foot, ensuring a snug fit and better weight distribution<br>Beneficial for correcting biomechanical issues like overpronation or supination<br>*Flat or minimal contour insoles*<br>Offer general cushioning without targeting specific support needs<br>Suitable for neutral feet or as temporary comfort solutions (Kumar & Sarangi, 2024)<br>Highly contoured insoles provide a precise fit that enhances stability and alignment, making them ideal for individuals with specific orthopedic needs. In contrast, flat or minimally contoured insoles prioritize basic comfort and flexibility, making them a good choice for everyday wear without corrective intervention. |

(continued)

**Table 3.1** (continued)

| |
|---|
| *Thickness and elevation*<br>The thickness of an insole affects cushioning, shock absorption, and how the foot fits inside the shoe. Choosing the right thickness depends on the intended use and footwear type:<br>*Thicker insoles*<br>Provide more cushioning and shock absorption.<br>May raise the foot too high in some footwear, affecting fitness and comfort.<br>*Thin insoles*<br>Fit better in tight or slim shoes but offer less cushioning (House et al., 2004).<br>Thicker insoles are often preferred for high-impact activities or individuals who require extra comfort and pressure relief. However, they may cause a snug fit in certain shoes. On the other hand, thin insoles work well for casual or dress shoes where space is limited but do not provide as much shock absorption. |
| *Tapering and slope*<br>The gradual tapering and slope of an insole influence weight transition during gait. A well-designed slope facilitates smoother movement and reduces strain on the foot. Different tapering and slope designs offer distinct benefits:<br>*Gradual taper*<br>Facilitates a smooth transition from heel to toe during walking or running<br>Reduces strain on the plantar fascia<br>*Abrupt slope*<br>May create pressure points or discomfort, especially for individuals with sensitive feet or poor biomechanics<br>A gradual taper provides a natural foot motion, promoting efficiency and reducing stress on the arch and forefoot. In contrast, an abrupt slope can disrupt weight distribution and lead to localized discomfort or pressure-related issues. |
| *Width and fit*<br>The width of an insole must match the user's foot and shoe width to ensure proper support, stability, and comfort. An ill-fitted insole can cause pressure points, discomfort, or misalignment. Different width options provide distinct benefits:<br>*Wide insoles*<br>Essential for individuals with wider feet to prevent pinching or misalignment<br>Enhances stability in wide shoes<br>*Narrow insoles*<br>Fit snugly in slim footwear but may not provide adequate support for wider feet.<br>Proper width selection ensures that the foot remains properly aligned within the shoe, reducing the risk of blisters, calluses, or foot fatigue. Wide insoles provide extra room for comfort, while narrow insoles ensure a secure fit in sleek or fashion-oriented footwear.<br>Each of these design elements plays a crucial role in determining the effectiveness of an insole. Understanding these factors helps in selecting or designing an insole that best suits an individual's foot structure, activity level, and specific needs. |

## 3.5 Insoles for Diabetic Foot

Diabetic foot problems occur due to complications arising from diabetes, primarily affecting nerves and blood vessels. The main causes include:

(i) Peripheral neuropathy: High blood sugar levels can cause nerve damage, leading to a loss of sensation in the feet. This makes it difficult to feel cuts, blisters, or injuries, which may go untreated and become infected.

(ii) Peripheral artery disease (PAD): Diabetes can lead to poor blood circulation in the feet. Reduced blood flow slows down wound healing and increases the risk of infection.
(iii) High blood sugar: Consistently high glucose levels can impair the body's ability to fight infections and delay the healing of any injuries or ulcers.
(iv) Foot deformities: Due to neuropathy and changes in foot shape, the pressure points in the foot may change, increasing the risk of developing sores and ulcers.
(v) Calluses and foot ulcers: Diabetic patients tend to develop calluses more easily, which can lead to skin breakdown and ulcers. These ulcers may get infected if not treated properly.

Diabetic insoles are specially designed foot orthotics that help prevent foot complications associated with diabetes, such as ulcers, blisters, and calluses. These insoles are intended to provide support, cushioning, and pressure distribution to minimize the risk of injury and improve overall foot health.

### 3.5.1 Features of Diabetic Insoles

(a) Pressure distribution: Diabetic insoles are designed to evenly distribute weight and reduce pressure points that could lead to ulcers [11].
(b) Cushioning: Extra cushioning helps reduce impact forces on the foot, preventing skin breakdown and reducing the risk of injuries [12].
(c) Arch support: Proper arch support is essential to maintain foot alignment, preventing abnormal pressure points [13].
(d) Moisture-wicking and breathable materials: Insoles are often made with materials that help keep the feet dry and reduce the risk of fungal infections.
(e) Seamless design: Diabetic insoles are made without seams or rough edges that can irritate the skin, preventing blisters.

## 3.6 Insoles for People with Foot Deformities or Conditions

### 3.6.1 Flat Feet

Flat feet, or pes planus, occur when the arch of the foot either fails to develop in childhood or collapses in adulthood. Causes include loose tendons in early childhood, genetic factors such as Ehlers-Danlos syndrome and Marfan syndrome, aging, injury, or illness that affects the tendons. In some cases, it may be due to tarsal coalition, where two or more bones in the foot grow together abnormally. Treatment may not be necessary if flat feet are painless. For painful flat feet, arch supports, proper footwear, and calf stretching may help. Severe cases may require surgery, such as tendon repair or joint fusion to restore arch structure. Flat feet occur when the arch of the foot collapses or is not prominent.

#### 3.6.1.1 Insole Design for Flat Feet

(a) Arch support: Insoles should have a contoured arch that provides medium to high support, depending on the severity of the flat foot. The goal is to offer corrective elevation to help distribute body weight evenly.
(b) Heel cup: A deep and firm heel cup to stabilize the foot and prevent overpronation.
(c) Cushioning: Extra cushioning in the heel and forefoot areas to provide comfort and shock absorption.

### 3.6.2 High Arches

High arches are often due to genetic factors or neurological conditions like Charcot-Marie-Tooth disease. The excessive arch places more weight on the ball and heel of the foot, which can lead to instability. Supportive shoes and custom orthotics help distribute weight more evenly. Physical therapy exercises and stretching can relieve discomfort, and surgical options are considered for severe cases. High arches create uneven weight distribution, often leading to excess pressure on the ball and heel of the foot.

#### 3.6.2.1 Insole Design for High Arches (Cavus Foot)

(a) Arch fill: Insoles should have a high arch fill that provides direct contact with the arch to distribute pressure more evenly.
(b) Heel and forefoot padding: Cushioning should be added to these areas to help alleviate excessive pressure points and provide better shock absorption.
(c) Flexible material: The insole should be flexible to adapt to the foot's shape while maintaining support for the arch.

### 3.6.3 Plantar Fasciitis

This condition involves inflammation of the plantar fascia, the band of tissue connecting the heel to the toes. Common causes include overuse, tight calf muscles, being overweight, or wearing poorly fitting shoes. Treatments include rest, ice packs, nonsteroidal anti-inflammatory drugs (NSAIDs), stretching exercises for the Achilles tendon and plantar fascia, and supportive footwear. Corticosteroid injections or surgery may be needed in severe cases. Plantar fasciitis is caused by inflammation of the plantar fascia ligament, leading to heel pain.

#### 3.6.3.1 Insole Design for Plantar Fasciitis

(a) Heel cushion: Ample cushioning under the heel to absorb shock and reduce the impact that aggravates the plantar fascia [14].

(b) Arch support: Moderate arch support to reduce strain on the plantar fascia, ensuring even weight distribution [15].
(c) Heel cup: A deep heel cup to cradle the heel, control motion, and provide stability [5].

### 3.6.4 Bunions

Bunions are bone deformities that develop at the joint of the big toe, often due to wearing tight or improperly fitting shoes, stress on the joint, or arthritis. Genetics can also play a role. Treatment includes wearing comfortable, well-fitting shoes, using protective pads, and taking pain relievers like ibuprofen. Severe bunions causing pain may require surgery. Bunions are bony bumps that form on the joint at the base of the big toe, often causing pain and discomfort.

#### 3.6.4.1 Insole Design for Bunions

(a) Metatarsal pad: A metatarsal pad to reduce pressure on the ball of the foot, which helps relieve bunion pain [16].
(b) Wide toe box: Insoles that work well in shoes with a wider toe box to accommodate the bunion and reduce pressure on the big toe joint [17].
(c) Soft materials: Use of soft, cushioning materials to alleviate friction and pressure points around the bunion [17].

## 3.7 Material Selection Criteria

The materials used in insole manufacturing can be categorized into three main groups, soft materials, rigid materials, and moisture-wicking materials, each serving distinct functional purposes. Table 3.2 presents the functions of various insole materials. Soft materials play a crucial role in enhancing comfort, cushioning, and shock absorption. These materials help distribute pressure evenly across the foot, reducing the risk of discomfort and fatigue. They are particularly beneficial for individuals with foot pain or high-impact activities. Rigid materials provide essential structural support, particularly in maintaining arch integrity and ensuring proper biomechanical alignment. These materials help control foot motion, prevent excessive pronation or supination, and improve overall stability.

Moisture-wicking materials are designed to manage perspiration by drawing moisture away from the skin and facilitating rapid evaporation. This feature helps keep feet dry, reducing the risk of blisters and fungal infections while enhancing overall foot hygiene. By selecting appropriate materials based on their functional properties, insoles can be optimized for specific user needs, whether for enhanced comfort, corrective support, or moisture control.

These materials can be selected or combined in insoles to provide tailored solutions for different needs such as comfort, shock absorption, or orthopedic support. These soft materials are chosen for their ability to cushion and protect diabetic feet,

**Table 3.2** Function of insole materials

| Type of materials | Name | Functions |
|---|---|---|
| Soft materials | EVA foam | Provides lightweight cushioning<br>Absorbs impact for high-energy activities<br>Adds support while retaining flexibility |
| | Memory foam | Offers custom-fit comfort by molding to the foot<br>Reduces pressure points, improving comfort for extended wear<br>Absorbs shock effectively, aiding in pain relief |
| | Gel inserts | Delivers targeted cushioning in high-impact zones (e.g., heel or forefoot)<br>Distributes pressure evenly across the foot<br>Enhances energy return during activities |
| | Silicone | Provides long-lasting cushioning<br>Reduces shear forces, which is beneficial for diabetic or sensitive feet<br>Suitable for extreme conditions due to temperature and moisture resistance |
| | Plastazote® foam | Often used for orthopedic insoles due to its moldability<br>Reduces friction and shear forces, protecting sensitive skin<br>Helps redistribute pressure for diabetic foot care |
| | Poron® | Offers superior cushioning and energy return<br>Maintains performance over time (non-compressive)<br>Provides antimicrobial properties to prevent odors |
| | Neoprene | Provides shock absorption and flexibility<br>Offers thermal insulation for warmth in cold environments<br>Durable for use in rugged activities or sports |
| | Cork | Offers firm support for arch and heel stability<br>Molds to the foot over time for customized support<br>Lightweight and eco-friendly |
| | Leather | Provides firm support and durability<br>Offers natural breathability and moisture-wicking<br>Ideal for dress shoe insoles due to aesthetics and function |
| | Urethane (Polyurethane) | Combines cushioning and support<br>Suitable for high-impact activities due to energy return<br>Often used for its balance of flexibility and durability |

(continued)

**Table 3.2** (continued)

| Type of materials | Name | Functions |
|---|---|---|
| Rigid materials | Carbon fiber | Provides rigid support for foot alignment and biomechanical correction<br>Reduces energy loss during motion, making it ideal for sports and high-performance insoles<br>Lightweight yet strong, adding structural integrity without bulk<br>Suitable for conditions requiring immobilization or limited foot movement (e.g., fractures, arthritis) |
| | Polypropylene (PP) | Offers moderate rigidity for arch and heel support<br>Commonly used in semi-rigid orthotic devices for biomechanical correction<br>Lightweight and cost-effective |
| | Polycarbonate (PC) | Provides rigid, durable support for demanding applications<br>Used in high-stress zones where structural integrity is essential<br>Offers flexibility to design for tailored biomechanical correction |
| | Acrylic (PMMA) | Primarily used in transparent or custom aesthetic orthotics<br>Offers rigidity for foot alignment with moderate cushioning |
| | Nylon (Polyamide) | Provides flexible support and durability<br>Used for semi-rigid orthotics that require some elasticity and shock absorption |

(continued)

**Table 3.2** (continued)

| Type of materials | Name | Functions |
|---|---|---|
| Moisture-wicking | Polyester fabrics (e.g., Coolmax®) | Wicks moisture away from the skin, keeping feet dry<br>Enhances airflow and reduces heat buildup<br>Durable and resistant to odor-causing bacteria |
| | Nylon fabrics | Provides a smooth, moisture-wicking surface layer<br>Lightweight and breathable for enhanced comfort<br>Often combined with antimicrobial treatments to reduce odors |
| | Merino wool | Absorbs moisture while remaining breathable, preventing sweaty or clammy feet<br>Naturally antimicrobial, reducing odor buildup<br>Provides temperature regulation (cool in summer, warm in winter) |
| | Bamboo fiber | Effectively wicks moisture and dries quickly<br>Naturally antibacterial and antifungal, reducing odors<br>Soft and comfortable for sensitive skin |
| | Microfiber | Enhances comfort with a soft touch<br>Improves moisture-wicking to keep feet dry<br>Acts as a durable upper layer for insoles<br>Wicks moisture efficiently to keep feet dry<br>Provides a smooth, soft surface that is comfortable for prolonged use<br>Often treated with antimicrobial finishes to prevent bacterial growth |
| | Polypropylene fiber (PP) | Acts as a hydrophobic layer, repelling moisture<br>Keeps insoles lightweight and dry, even in high-sweat environments<br>Commonly used as a base layer for moisture-wicking fabrics |
| | Tencel® (Lyocell) | Draws moisture away from the foot for a dry feeling<br>Environmentally friendly and biodegradable<br>Soft and gentle on the skin, ideal for sensitive users |
| | Cotton (treated for moisture-wicking) | Absorbs sweat effectively when treated for quicker drying<br>Provides a soft and breathable surface<br>May include antimicrobial treatments to combat odor |
| | Gore-Tex® linings | Acts as a waterproof yet breathable layer<br>Allows moisture vapor to escape while preventing external water ingress<br>Ideal for outdoor or athletic applications |

prevent ulcers, reduce pressure points, and manage moisture, all of which are critical in minimizing the risks associated with diabetic foot complications. When designing diabetic insoles, the material selection must prioritize foot protection, pressure relief, moisture control, and comfort to prevent complications like ulcers, blisters, or infections. Diabetic patients, especially those with neuropathy, are at high risk for foot injuries due to reduced sensation and circulation, so the insole materials must provide cushioning, pressure redistribution, and support without causing friction or irritation. The previous study showed that the additional multi-foam layer on top of conventional materials (i.e., platozote and microcellular rubber) provided better plantar pressure distribution in diabetic feet with neuropathy [16].

The rigid materials are chosen for structural support: maintains arch support and biomechanical alignment and prevents overpronation or supination. Another way there has function to weight reduction: Many rigid materials are lightweight, improving comfort without sacrificing strength. They have corrective and protective roles: used for medical-grade orthotics to address foot deformities or injuries and protects feet from excessive movement in conditions like plantar fasciitis or metatarsalgia. Due to the properties of the material, when in the insole, it will make insoles durable: resistant to wear and deformation, ensuring long-lasting performance. Rigid materials are typically combined with softer layers (e.g., foams or gels) to balance comfort and support. Their selection depends on the specific requirements of the user, activity level, and medical needs. Rigid materials like carbon fiber reduce energy loss, aiding active users.

Moisture-wicking materials are often combined with cushioning and structural layers in insoles for a comprehensive performance solution. There is key to keep feet dry by pulling sweat away from the skin and allowing it to evaporate quickly and helps maintain a cool and comfortable foot environment, reducing overheating. Many materials include antimicrobial properties to minimize bacterial growth and odors. It reduces friction and hotspots caused by sweat, enhancing comfort during prolonged wear or athletic activities, and resistant to repeated washing and prolonged use without losing functionality.

## 3.8 Manufacturing Techniques

Making a custom-made insole involves several steps depending on the type of insole. Insoles can be handmade or made with computer-aided design/computer-aided manufacturing (CAD/CAM) or rapid prototyping techniques. There are several manufacturing techniques for insole fabrication including conventional fabrication, digitalized manufacturing, subtractive manufacturing, and additive manufacturing.

### 3.8.1 Conventional Technique

In daily practice of a prostheses and orthoses unit, an orthotist performs this task manually with the equipment in the workshop. This technique requires a skill orthotist and time consume. There are several steps required for this technique from casting foot shapes to fitting insoles. The insole fabricated using this conventional method is known as "a custom-made insole."

- **Step1: Casting Foot Shape**
  Patient has to step on the foam impression box to acquire the foot geometry by starting with the heel and moving toward the toes. The foot should be dry and clean for a clear impression. It is necessary to ensure that the foot is in a neutral position to capture a natural arch and entire foot length and width. It is important to apply even pressure over the entire foot to make a clear and deep impression. Pressing on key areas, including the heel, arch, and toes, to ensure the contours of the foot are captured accurately. The contours of the foot are cast in the foam. The excessive pressure while making the contours can distort the shape. The front part cast toes are smoothed by compressing the front part creating a smooth extension. The foot measurement note should be put on the foam impression box for reference, that is, length and width. After smoothing, the molds for the insole are ready to perform a foot model casting.
  Next step is to perform the plaster foot model casting. The foam impression box has to be placed on the stable and flat surface to ensure it does not move while pouring the plaster. Plaster of Paris is mixed with water in a container and consistently stirred to make the mixture thick enough to hold shape but still pourable. It should be careful to avoid air bubbles in the plaster while mixing by stirring slowly and thoroughly. The plaster mixture is carefully poured into the foam impression box by starting from the heel and gradually moves to the front as shown in Fig. 3.2. It is important to make sure that the entire footprint is filled without gaps. Furthermore, a gently knock on the side of foam box can be done to release air bubbles that might be trapped in the plaster. If there are trapped bubbles in the plaster the final plaster model can be distorted. When pouring plaster mixture, the depth should capture the full depth of the foot impression in the foam to ensure the model includes the heel, arch, ball, and toe contours. The surface level of the plaster is smoothed with the foam impression box's edge to create a stable base of the model. Then, the plaster has to be cured. Usually, the curing time is 30 to 60 minutes depending on the type of plaster and environmental conditions. To prevent cracking or shifting of plaster cast, the foam impression box should not be moved during this curing period. When the plaster is fully hardened, the plaster model is lifted out of the foam impression box. In case an additional cast is needed, the foam impression should not be damaged. After taking the model out of the foam impression box, the model has to be inspected to ensure it accurately reflects the foot's contours. Trimming the excess plaster around the edges is required to smooth out the base.
- **Step 2: Forming Insole**

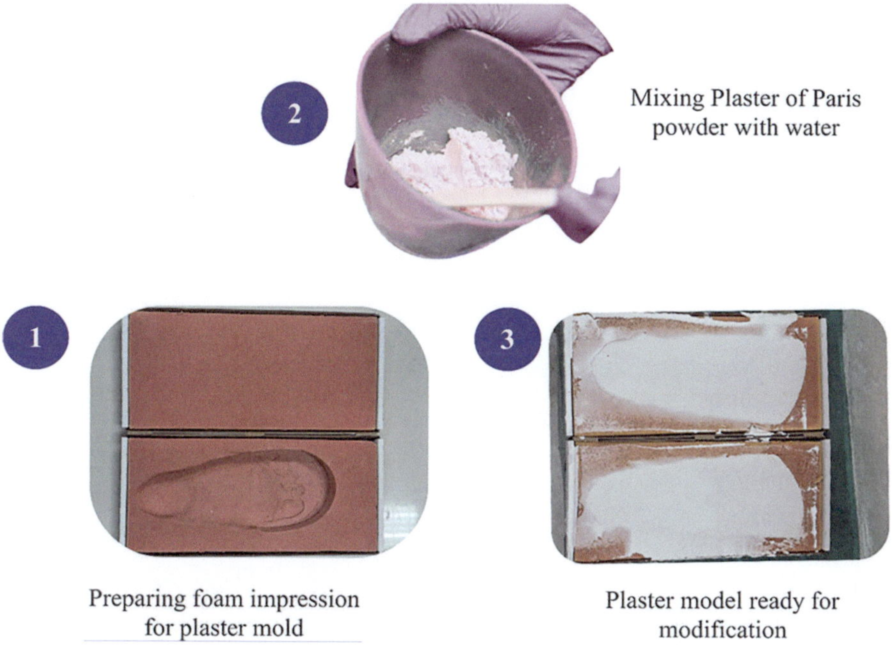


**Fig. 3.2** Making a foot model using plaster mixture pouring in the foam box

As mentioned in the previous section about the materials, the proper materials should be selected regarding the purpose of insoles such as desired support, flexibility, and cushioning. Generally, thermoplastic or ethylene vinyl acetate (EVA) sheet is used for the insole. The thermoplastic sheet was heated by putting it in a low-temperature oven until it becomes flexible. Material should be warm enough and uniformly heated to avoid uneven deformation. The heated sheet is placed over the plaster foot model and carefully pressed down to capture the contours of the foot model. It is necessary to press firmly along the arch, heel cup, and other areas that require extra support to ensure good fitness (Fig. 3.3). Material is then cooled and hardened while it is on the foot model to retain the molded shape. In addition, for pressing the thermoplastic sheet on the plaster model, it can use the vacuum mold to capture the contour and firmly press. Excess material along the edges of the insole must be trimmed out following the shape of the foot model.

- **Step3: Polishing and Fitting Insoles**
  Any rough or sharp edges around the insole should be smoothed by using sandpaper or grinding machine as shown in Fig. 3.4. Fine-grit sandpaper is used to polish the areas that feel rough or uncomfortable under foot. In some cases, using an edge smoother or beveling tool is performed to smooth the edges for more comfort and good-looking. In addition, to make a professional look, a top cover can be put on the insole using leather or foam. The top cover material is glued on the top surface with adhesive and firmly pressed to avoid the air bubbles. Using

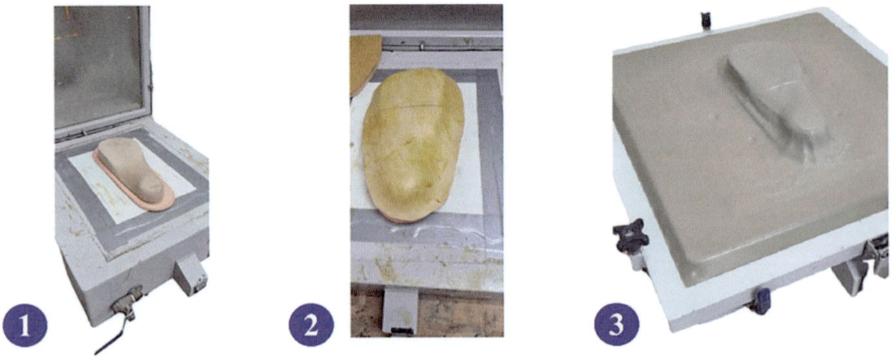


**Fig. 3.3** Forming insoles using thermoplastic sheet for hot pressing around the foot model

**Fig. 3.4** Polishing and smoothing an insole using a grinding machine

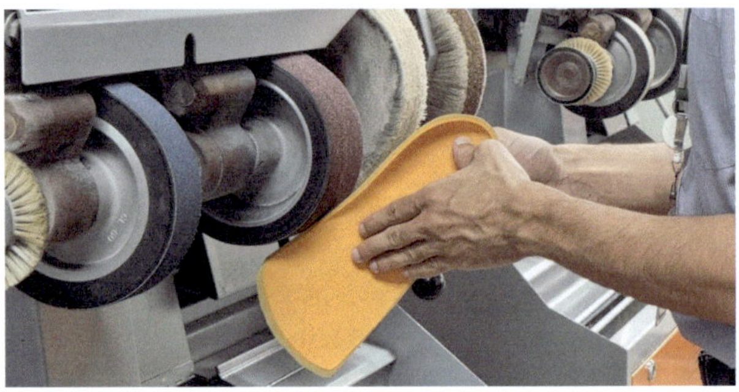

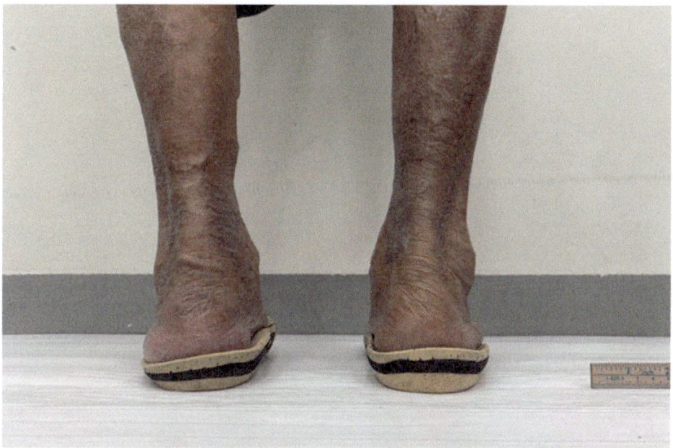

**Fig. 3.5** Insole checking and fitting with patient's foot

a soft cloth or microfiber towel to remove dust from sanding or grinding. The insole is checked by putting it underneath the patient's foot and placing the insole inside the shoe (Fig. 3.5). It is necessary to ensure that the patient feels comfortable, and the insole lies flat without shifting or rubbing.

### 3.8.2 Digitalized Manufacturing

Compared to a conventional practice for a customized insole, using digital technology can reduce laborious work, lower manufacturing waste and save time. Furthermore, it can enhance the effectiveness of reproducing the insole. To acquire the foot shape, a three-dimensional (3D) scanner is used either a handheld scanner or a stationary scanner as shown in Fig. 3.6. The foot model is reconstructed and pre-processed in the scanner software or compatible software (e.g., EXScan Pro, Solid Edge SHINING 3D Edition, Geomagic Qualify) before exporting as a Polygon (PLY) or Standard Tessellation Language or Standard Triangulation Language (STL) file formats for the next step which is an insole design [18]. The PLY format commonly stores three-dimensional data from 3D scanners. The STL format represents only the surface geometry of a three-dimensional object.

The customized insole is designed to fit with the 3D foot geometry using computer-aided design (CAD) software both commercial (e.g., SolidWorks, Fusion 360, SpaceClaim) and free (e.g., Blender and EasyCAD) software. Furthermore, 3D printed orthosis design software like MediACE3D, OrthoModel Pro, and nTopology are available for insole design. The shape and thickness of the insole are adjusted and finalized in this software. Furthermore, the information of foot plantar pressure distribution or plantar pressure mapping during standing and walking is taken into consideration for designing an insole in terms of high-pressure and low-pressure locations [19]. The 3D geometry of insoles is saved in the STL format for insole manufacturing.

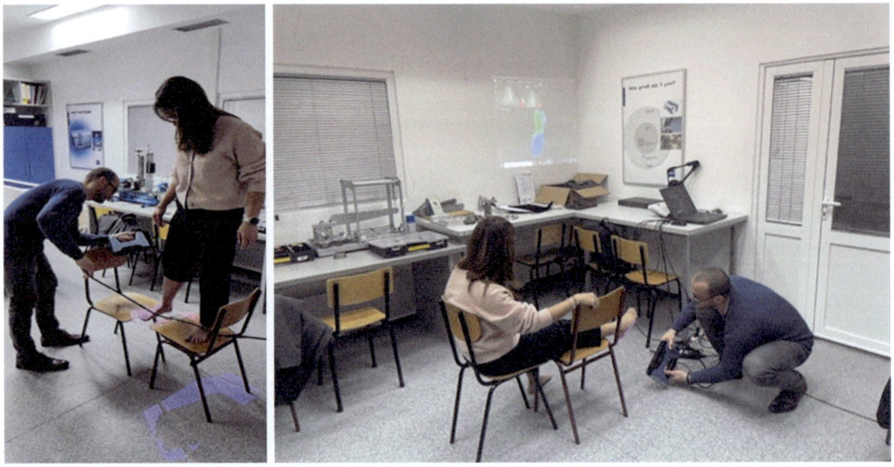

**Fig. 3.6** Scanning the foot using 3D scanner to obtain foot shape

### 3.8.3 Subtractive Manufacturing Techniques

Subtractive manufacturing is a method to remove material from a solid block or sheet to shape an object. There are several subtractive manufacturing techniques such as computer numerical control (CNC) milling, laser cutting, or manual carving. An insole can be fabricated using these techniques by preparing the material blocks or sheets that fit to the CNC machine. Ethylene vinyl acetate (EVA) foam and polyurethane foam (PU) are common materials used for insole milling. Computer-aided manufacturing (CAM) software is used to generate toolpaths for material removal based on the 3D geometry of insoles which is saved in the STL format. An important concern for subtractive manufacturing techniques is waste from material removal. Therefore, the toolpath optimization is required to reduce waste. It is also necessary to choose cutting tools, cutting speed, and feed rate based on selected materials. For a material block, CNC milling cuts it into the insole shape and contours layer by layer. Several studies reported the optimal parameters with respect to a flat surface for CNC milling [20]. The effective offloading of the foot to prevent foot ulcers depends on the hardness of the material and dimension accuracy of the insoles which are strongly dependent on the machining process. The surface quality of insoles using CNC milling on different surface hardness of EVA foam was studied and found that the EVA foam with a surface hardness of 20–35 HRC was suitable material insoles and able to be manufactured through CNC milling [20]. For thin material, laser cutting is preferable for precise shape cutting. After milling, it is necessary to adjust if the surface of insole has roughness by using sandpaper or grinding machine. There are several drawbacks of subtractive manufacturing such as material waste, lack of flexibility to alternate materials in different areas, and no gain access to the inside of object (3D printing of functional anatomical insoles).

### 3.8.4 Additive Manufacturing Techniques

Additive manufacturing, commonly known as 3D printing, is a method of making three-dimensional objects from a digital model by adding layer by layer using different manufacturing techniques such as material extrusion, vat photopolymerization, powder bed fusion, and material jetting. Additive manufacturing has several benefits compared to subtractive manufacturing such as lower waste, no dust, lower cost of material, and lesser labor. The most popular and affordable 3D printing is fused deposition modeling (FDM). This technique takes a polymer-based filament and extrudes it through a heated nozzle, which melts the material and deposits it in 2D layers on the heated platform to stack it and create a 3D part. There are many commercial polymer-based filaments which are used with FDM. It is like a subtractive manufacturing that starts from the insole's STL format produced from CAD software [21]. Then the STL file is imported to the 3D slicer software to render the 3D object before printing. Many 3D slicer software is open source for the 3D printer such as PrusaSlicer, Cura, Slic3r, IdeaMaker, Simplify 3D, and Blender. Figure 3.7 shows the flat insole rendered in ideaMaker 5.14 for Raise3D Pro2 Plus. Within the slicer software, there are many settings that can be changed including printing speed, infill pattern, infill density, nozzle temperature, cooldown, etc. One important setting parameter for printing is an infill pattern which has many patterns such as cubic, gyroid, honeycomb, triangle, and grid. Figure 3.8 shows 3D printed specimens with different infill patterns and infill densities. In the slicer software, it can calculate the material usage and time of production for the estimated product price. The printing time depends on the size, structure, infill pattern, infill density, and material filament. During printing process, the printer's nozzle moves in x- and y-directions while the hot plate moves in the z-direction as shown in Fig. 3.9. After printing, the insoles are needed to perform a post-processing and finishing.

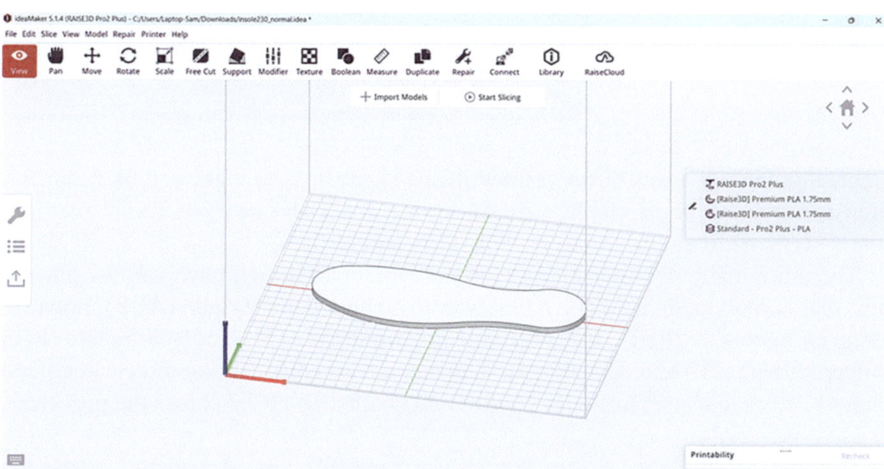


**Fig. 3.7** The display of ideaMaker 5.14 for the Raise3D Pro2 Plus 3D printer

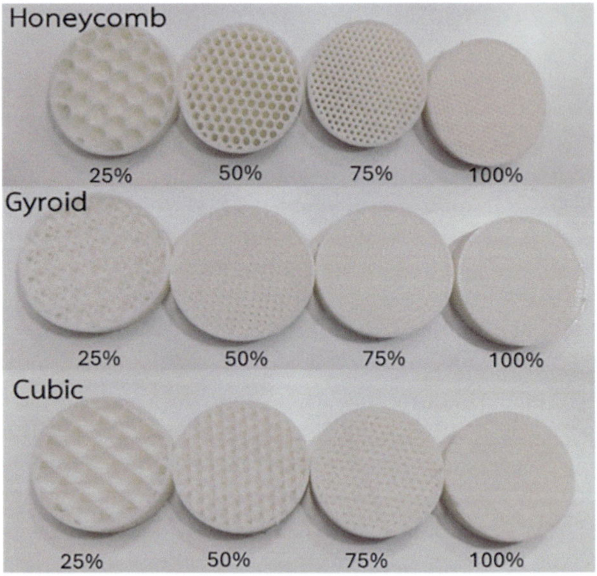


**Fig. 3.8** Infill patterns and infill densities of printed specimens

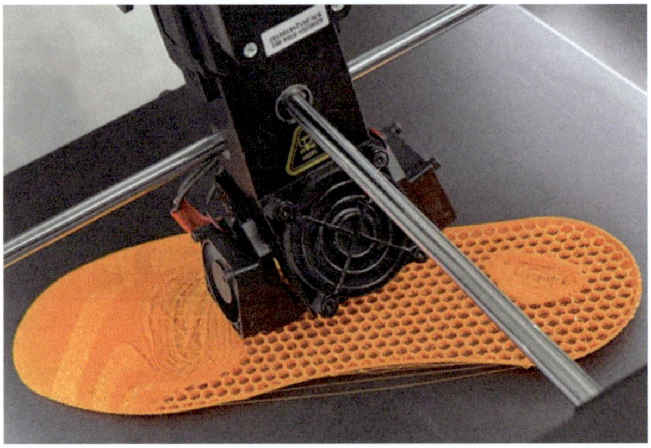

**Fig. 3.9** Printing nozzle moves in the x-y plane to print the insole on the hot plate

Generally, the top cover of the printed insole is required to make it look beautiful, high quality, and comfortable. The top cover materials are EVA foam, memory foam, urethane foam, mesh fabric, TPU film, and leather.

There are many polymer-based materials for FDM which have various properties, that is, polylactic acid (PLA), acrylonitrile butadiene styrene (ABS), polyethylene terephthalate (PET), thermoplastic polyurethane (TPU), polycarbonate (PC), polypropylene (PP), etc. Usually, these materials are graded along three categories: process, mechanical performance, and visual quality. Table 3.3 shows the properties of FDM materials.

Furthermore, there are several studies using reinforcing materials to increase the thermal stability and mechanical properties of FDM materials [22–25]. Carbon fiber is one of the reinforce materials to create polymer composites due to its light weight,

**Table 3.3** Material properties of printing filaments

| Properties | ABS | TPU | PLA | PET | PC | PVA | PP | Nylon |
|---|---|---|---|---|---|---|---|---|
| Maximum service temperature (°C) | 98 | 60–74 | 52 | 73 | 121 | 75 | 100 | 80–95 |
| Extruder temperature (°C) | 220–250 | 225–245 | 190–220 | 230–250 | 260–310 | 185–200 | 220–250 | 220–270 |
| Bed temperature (°C) | 95–110 | 45–60 | 45–60 | 75–90 | 80–120 | 45–60 | 85–100 | 70–90 |
| Density (g/cm$^3$) | 1.04 | 1.19–1.23 | 1.24 | 1.23 | 1.2 | 1.23 | 0.9 | 1.06–1.14 |
| Ultimate strength (MPa) | 40 | 26–43 | 65 | 53 | 72 | 78 | 32 | 40–85 |
| Stiffness | Moderate | Low | High | Moderate | Moderate | Low | Low | Moderate |
| Durability | High | High | Low | High | Very high | Moderate | High | Very high |
| Impact resistant | ✓ | – | – | – | ✓ | – | – | ✓ |
| Heat resistant | ✓ | – | – | – | ✓ | – | ✓ | ✓ |
| Chemical resistant | – | – | – | ✓ | – | – | – | – |
| Fatigue resistant | – | ✓ | – | ✓ | ✓ | ✓ | ✓ | ✓ |
| Visual quality | Moderate | Low | High | Moderate | Moderate | Low | High | Moderate |

mechanical strength, and thermal stability [26]. However, carbon fiber has a drawback which is it is not biodegradable. Not only carbon fiber but glass fiber and aramid fiber are also used as reinforce materials to increase stiffness and high-impact resistance.

## 3.9 Integration of AI into Insole Design and Customization

Artificial intelligence (AI) has become a new wave of technology which can assist and perform tasks with less human operation. Nowadays, AI has been widely used in many fields such as language translation and speech recognition, autonomous vehicles, drug discovery and development, personalized treatment plans, and product and industrial design, including insole design and fabrication. For example, using AI-driven approaches to customize a diabetic shoe insole was implemented by enhancing wound area identification and measurement, detecting elevated pressure area on the foot and identifying needed pressure offloading site [27]. To design and prescribe a customized insole, it is necessary to know the plantar pressure distribution, foot stability, arch index, and individual needs. This data can be efficiently processed by using machine learning to classify, determine, and propose the best problem-solution fit. Several machine learning classifiers, that is, support vector machine, k-nearest neighbor, and Naïve Bayes, were used to classify the features extracted from spatiotemporal and morphological information that the results can be aided in the design of pressure insoles for occupational safety [28]. It was shown that using AI with foot scan data provided effective decision-making for designers. However, the accuracy of AI prediction depends on the number of input parameters [29]. Data-driven custom-made footwear concepts can effectively reduce peak plantar pressures at metatarsal head area in diabetic patients [30]. Additionally, the advantages of using AI in the insole design are informative key features of the insole design which match the foot problems. For example, in Box 3.1, a generative AI can provide information and considerations for making an insole for high arch feet such as arch support, metatarsal support, heel cushioning, and material composition. A generative AI can provide a 3D visual of the insole in its answers for better understanding. Therefore, by integrating AI into insole design and customization, it can enhance more personalization, efficiency, and effectiveness which are benefits to customers and patients.

**Box 3.1: Generative AI for Insole Design (Created with ChatGPT)**

**Prompt:** If a patient has a high arch foot, please design a suitable insole for this patient.

**Answer by ChatGPT:** For a patient with high-arched feet (pes cavus), the insole should provide proper support, cushioning, and pressure redistribution. Below is a suitable insole design for such a condition:

**Key Features of the Insole Design**

1. Arch Support
   - A well-contoured, high arch support to fill the gap under the foot
   - Should provide firm but cushioned support to prevent excessive pressure on the heel and forefoot
2. Metatarsal Support (Forefoot Cushioning)
   - A metatarsal pad to help distribute pressure evenly across the ball of the foot
   - Reduces forefoot pain and risk of metatarsalgia
3. Heel Cushioning
   - Extra shock-absorbing padding in the heel area to reduce impact forces
   - Helps prevent heel pain, especially if the patient has a tendency for plantar fasciitis
4. Material Composition
   - EVA foam base for lightweight yet durable support
   - Gel or poron inserts in the heel and forefoot for shock absorption
   - Breathable top layer to prevent excessive moisture buildup
5. Deep Heel Cup
   - Helps stabilize the heel and prevent excessive rolling (supination)
   - Improves overall foot alignment
6. Customizable Design
   - If the patient has lateral instability, slight posting on the lateral side to prevent excessive supination
   - Cutouts for pressure relief in specific areas if the patient has calluses or pain points

**Additional Considerations**

- Custom orthotics: If the patient has severe symptoms, a custom orthotic made from a foot mold would be ideal.
- Shoe compatibility: The insole should fit well in the patient's footwear (running shoes, casual shoes, or orthopedic footwear).
- Activity level: If the patient is an athlete, a more rigid carbon fiber or TPU-reinforced arch may be beneficial.

## References


1. Nagano H, Begg RK. Shoe-insole technology for injury prevention in walking. Sensors (Basel, Switzerland). 2018;18(5):E1468.
2. Bus SA, Busch-Westbroek TE, Pulles J, van Dun T, Szabo G, Lacorte DH, et al. Pressure-relieving effect of different insole top covers in people with diabetes at high risk of foot ulceration. Sensors (Basel, Switzerland). 2024;24(17):5549.
3. Nouman M, Leelasamran W, Chatpun S. Effectiveness of total contact orthosis for plantar pressure redistribution in neuropathic diabetic patients during different walking activities. Foot Ankle Int. 2017;38(8):901–8.
4. Zhang J, Lu S, Yang Y, Liu Y, Guo Y, Wang H. Efficacy of auxetic lattice structured shoe sole in advancing footwear comfort-from the perspective of plantar pressure and contact area. Front Public Health. 2024;12:1412518.
5. Li L, Yang L, Yu F, Shi J, Zhu L, Yang X, et al. 3D printing individualized heel cup for improving the self-reported pain of plantar fasciitis. J Transl Med. 2018;16(1):167.
6. Huang YP, Peng HT, Wang X, Chen ZR, Song CY. The arch support insoles show benefits to people with flatfoot on stance time, cadence, plantar pressure and contact area. PLoS One. 2020;15(8):e0237382.
7. Zhao X, Wang M, Fekete G, Baker JS, Wiltshire H, Gu Y. Analyzing the effect of an arch support functional insole on walking and jogging in young, healthy females. Technol Health Care. 2021;29(6):1141–51.
8. Hastings MK, Mueller MJ, Pilgram TK, Lott DJ, Commean PK, Johnson JE. Effect of metatarsal pad placement on plantar pressure in people with diabetes mellitus and peripheral neuropathy. Foot Ankle Int. 2007;28(1):84–8.
9. Männikkö K, Sahlman J. The effect of metatarsal padding on pain and functional ability in metatarsalgia. Scand J Surg. 2017;106(4):332–7.
10. Brunzini A, Mandolini M, Germani M, Nester C, Williams A. A knowledge-based and multi-user platform for prescribing custom-made insoles; 2018. p. 2597–608.
11. Masłowska-Lipowicz I, Adamczyk M, Gajewski R, Paruzel T, Lawinska K, Rostocki A. Footwear for diabetics—structural and material elements for the prevention and alleviation of foot lessions. Fibres Text East Eur. 2024;32:1–14.
12. Ren Y, Wang H, Song X, Wu Y, Lyu Y, Zeng W. Advancements in diabetic foot insoles: a comprehensive review of design, manufacturing, and performance evaluation. Front Bioeng Biotechnol. 2024;12:1394758.
13. Bianchi I, Forcellese A, Simoncini M, Vita A. Mechanical characterization and sustainability assessment of recycled EVA for footwears. Int J Adv Manuf Technol. 2023;126:1–12.
14. Oliveira HA, Jones A, Moreira E, Jennings F, Natour J. Effectiveness of total contact insoles in patients with plantar fasciitis. J Rheumatol. 2015;42(5):870–8.
15. Roxas M. Plantar fasciitis: diagnosis and therapeutic considerations. Altern Med Rev. 2005;10(2):83–93.
16. Nouman M, Dissaneewate T, Leelasamran W, Chatpun S. The insole materials influence the plantar pressure distributions in diabetic foot with neuropathy during different walking activities. Gait Posture. 2019;74:154–61.
17. Park CH, Chang MC. Forefoot disorders and conservative treatment. J Yeungnam Med Sci. 2019;36(2):92–8.
18. Spahiu T, Shehi E, Galantucci L, Kaçani J, Piperi E. 3D low cost scanning systems for extracting foot dimensions 2015.
19. Jonnala UK, Sankineni R, Ravi KY. Design and development of fused deposition modeling (FDM) 3D-printed orthotic insole by using gyroid structure. J Mech Behav Biomed Mater. 2023;145:106005.
20. Anggoro PW, Bawono B, Jamari J, Tauviqirrahman M, Bayuseno A. Advanced design and manufacturing of custom orthotics insoles based on hybrid Taguchi-response surface method. Heliyon. 2021;7:e06481.

21. Wang K, Lu C, Ye R, He W, Wei X, Li Y, et al. Research and development of 3D printing orthotic insoles and preliminary treatment of leg length discrepancy patients. Technol Health Care. 2020;28(6):615–24.
22. Blanco I, Cicala G, Recca G, Tosto C. Specific heat capacity and thermal conductivity measurements of PLA-based 3D-printed parts with milled carbon fiber reinforcement. Entropy. 2022;24:654.
23. Jamadi AH, Razali N, Petrů M, Taha MM, Muhammad N, Ilyas RA. Effect of chemically treated kenaf fibre on mechanical and thermal properties of PLA composites prepared through fused deposition modeling (FDM). Polymers. 2021;13(19):3299.
24. Papa I, Silvestri AT, Ricciardi MR, Lopresto V, Squillace A. Effect of fibre orientation on novel continuous 3D-printed fibre-reinforced composites. Polymers. 2021;13(15):2524.
25. Usun A, Gümrük R. The mechanical performance of the 3D printed composites produced with continuous carbon fiber reinforced filaments obtained via melt impregnation. Addit Manuf. 2021;46:102112.
26. Sha J, Dai J, Li J, Wei ZQ, Hausherr JM, Krenkel W. Influence of thermal treatment on thermo-mechanical stability and surface composition of carbon fiber. Appl Surf Sci. 2013;274:89–94.
27. Ariyasinghe N, Dahanayake U, Samarasinghe K, Samarakoon D, Krishara J, Weerathunga I. Enhancing diabetic shoe insole customization with AI-driven approaches; 2023. p. 149–54.
28. O'Sullivan P, Menolotto M, Visentin A, O'Flynn B, Komaris S. AI-based task classification with pressure insoles for occupational safety. IEEE Access. 2024;12:21347–57.
29. Khaing H, Chaiprapat S, Rungsri T, Yuangyai C, Jirasatitsin S, Chaiprapat S. Automated design of affordable modular custom insoles by multi-classification algorithms. Manage Syst Prod Eng. 2021;29:151–61.
30. Zwaferink JBJ, Custers W, Paardekooper I, Berendsen HA, Bus SA. Optimizing footwear for the diabetic foot: data-driven custom-made footwear concepts and their effect on pressure relief to prevent diabetic foot ulceration. PLoS One. 2020;15(4):e0224010.

# Clinical Evaluation and Prescription of Insoles

4

Muhammad Nouman and Surapong Chatpun

## 4.1 Patient Assessment for Insole Prescription

Diabetic neuropathy leads to loss of protective sensation and altered foot biomechanics, placing patients at high risk for plantar foot ulceration and re-ulceration. Customized foot insoles are prescribed to reduce and redistribute the abnormal plantar pressure, absorb shock, and protect vulnerable foot regions. Insoles aim to reduce abnormal ground reaction force to the foot and lover limb, thereby preventing ulcer formation. By conforming to the plantar surface, insoles distribute load over a larger area and offload bony prominences, which reduces peak plantar pressure and the risk of tissue breakdown. In practice, insoles may be used prophylactically in high-risk patients and therapeutically in those with active or healing ulcers. Their intended clinical effects include lowering peak plantar pressure 20–30% (or more with specialized design) and optimizing pressure distribution during gait. While cushioning materials like EVA and Poron attenuate impact, total-contact designs enable broad loading distribution. Thus, the primary purpose of insoles in diabetic neuropathy is ulcer prevention and foot preservation by pressure offloading techniques.

A thorough diabetic foot examination is essential to guide insole prescription. Clinicians should systematically screen for neuropathy, vascular status, and deformities. The key components that should be considered for screening diabetic foot

M. Nouman (✉)
Sirindhorn School of Prosthetics and Orthotics, Faculty of Medicine, Siriraj Hospital, Mahidol University, Bangkok, Thailand
e-mail: muhammad.nou@mahidol.ac.th

S. Chatpun
Department of Biomedical Sciences and Biomedical Engineering, Faculty of Medicine, Prince of Songkla University, Songkhla, Thailand



M. Nouman, S. Chatpun (eds.), *A Comprehensive Guide to Insole-Based Approaches for Diabetic Foot Complications*,
https://doi.org/10.1007/978-981-95-0656-9_4

include neurological testing, vascular assessment, and foot inspection. Neurological testing uses a 10-gram Semmes-Weinstein monofilament to assess protective sensation, with the inability to perceive pressure indicating neuropathy. Vibration testing with a 128 Hz tuning fork or biothesiometer is also used. Loss of sensation on two or more sites signifies high ulceration risk. Moreover, vascular assessment is conducted by palpating foot pulses and measuring ankle-brachial index (ABI) if indicated ABI <0.90 suggests cardiovascular risk. Another important aspect is to examine skin (calluses, ulcers, infections), nails, joint deformities (hammertoes, Charcot), and gait. Rigid deformities (claw toes, rocker bottom foot) localized high plantar stresses (Fig. 4.1).

Risk stratification in diabetic foot care, used by the International Working Group on the Diabetic Foot (IWGDF) and the International Diabetes Federation (IDF), categorizes patients from low to high risk of ulceration based on sensory loss, deformity, and vascular disease. In general, any patient with loss of protective sensation or deformity is considered at risk and requires preventive measures. Guidelines strongly recommend well-fitted therapeutic shoes and custom insoles for at-risk feet. In particular, if deformities or pre-ulcerative signs present, prescribing custom therapeutic footwear or insoles is indicated. Moreover, to reduce recurrent plantar ulcers, footwear must demonstrably offload pressure: the IWGDF defines effective therapeutic footwear as achieving ~30% reduction in plantar peak pressure versus standard shoes [1]. Clinical decision-making thus integrates the patients' neuropathic status, vascular health, biomechanical deformities, and ulcer history to determine the needs, types, and urgency of insole intervention.

## 4.2 Custom vs. Prefabricated Insoles

To prescribe insoles for diabetic feet, it is varied widely in design, materials, and intended clinical outcomes. Broadly, insoles can be classified into prefabricated insoles, custom-made insoles, or total contact insoles (Fig. 4.2). Custom-made insoles, often fabricated using manual molding or CAD/CAM techniques, are specifically tailored to match the patient's unique foot morphology and foot condition. Custom-made insoles provide maximal surface contact, effectively redistributing plantar pressure to minimize localized high-pressure zones. These insoles are integral for patients with moderate to severe neuropathy and those with previous ulcerations. The classification of insoles can be done based on diabetic foot severity. Low-risk patients (mild neuropathy and no foot deformities) require prefabricated insoles with basic cushioning and minimal customization and are typically sufficient to reduce pressure peaks moderately. These insoles are designed to offer cushioning and minimal arch support. Prefabricated insoles may incorporate soft multi-density layers and metatarsal pads but are limited in customization. However, custom-made insoles are designed based on positive mold or 3D scan of the patient's foot, ensuring precise contouring to foot anatomy.

Custom-made insole provides substantial offloading by increasing total contact area and incorporating additional features (metatarsal pads, metatarsal bar, arch

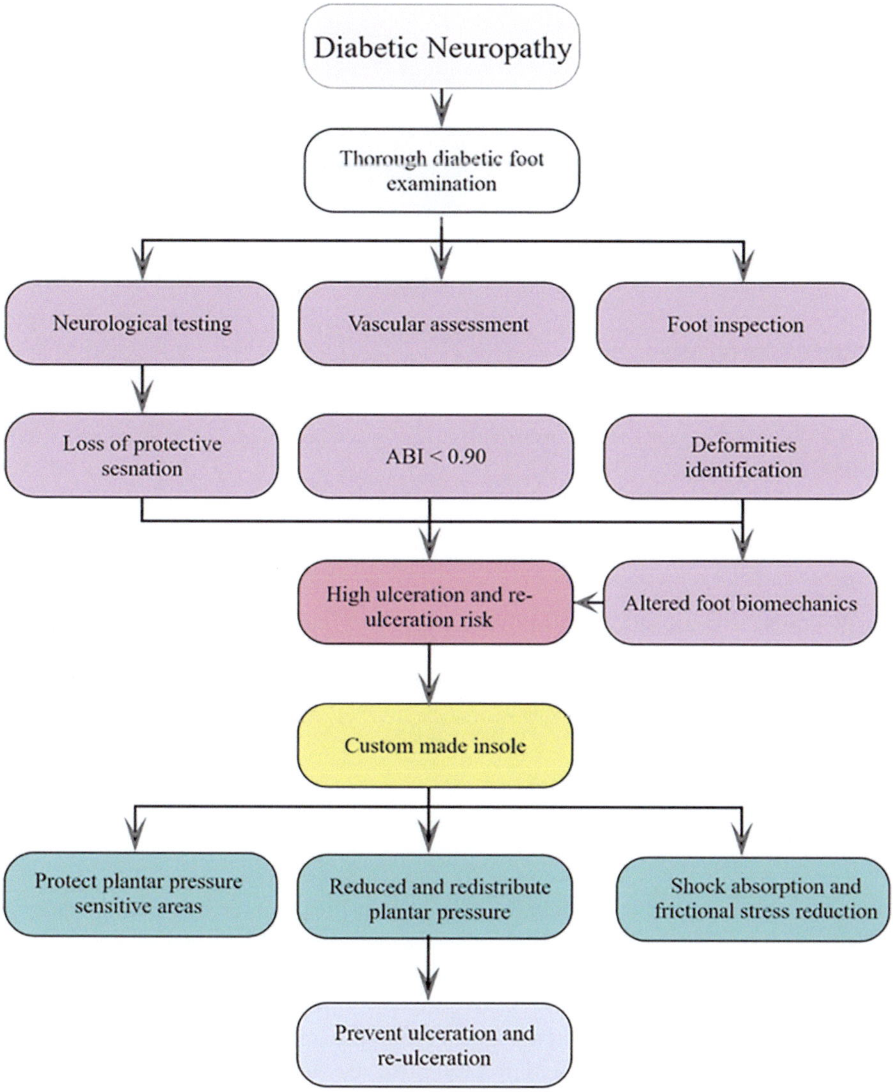


**Fig. 4.1** Flowchart of patient assessment for insole prescription; initial evaluation includes history and comprehensive foot exam

support, or cutouts for vulnerable regions) to further offloading by increasing total contact area. Custom-made and prefabricated insoles are ideal for moderate-risk patients with neuropathy and mild to moderate foot deformities to redistribute pressure accurately and stabilize foot structure. Evidence on prefabricated and custom-made insoles are mixed in terms of pressure distribution in low-risk foot. A randomized controlled trial found no significant differences in peak plantar pressure reduction between a custom-made insole and a prefabricated insole. The

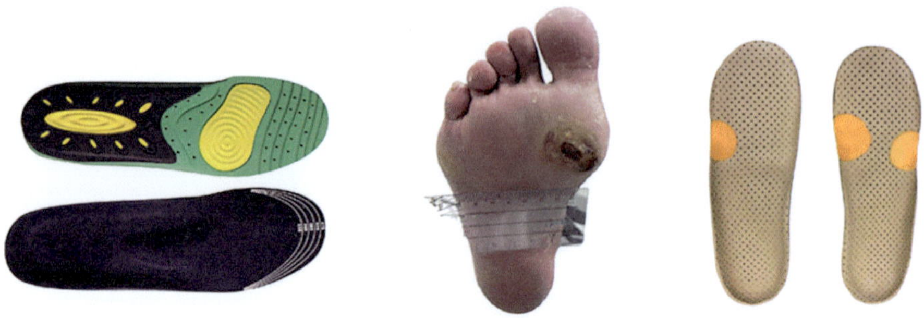


**Fig. 4.2** Prefabricated insoles and prescribed custom-made insole for diabetic foot with callus and ulceration

**Table 4.1** The pros and cons between custom-made insoles and prefabricated insoles

| | Pros | Cons |
|---|---|---|
| Custom-made insoles | Personalization/ perfect fit<br>Unlimited modifications<br>Suitable for any foot shape, regardless of deformity<br>Durability and longevity | Cost<br>Time-consuming |
| Prefabricated insoles | Cost-effective<br>Convenience<br>Adequate for mild conditions<br>No required casting | Limited customization<br>Durability<br>Fit issues |

custom-made insole did produce slightly better forefoot pressure-time integral offloading but at substantially higher cost. Patient-reported foot health and quality-of-life measures were similar between groups. However, clinicians recommend custom-made insoles to be more effective for ulcer prevention and better offloading of abnormal peak plantar pressure [2, 3]. Table 4.1 summarizes the pros and cons between custom-made insoles and prefabricated insoles.

Beyond fabrication mode, insoles are also classified as functional (biomechanical or correction of structural deformities) and accommodative (accommodate structural deformities) insoles. Functional insoles use firm arch supports, heel lifts, or posts to correct alignment and offload specific areas, whereas accommodative insoles focus on soft materials (Poron or Plastazote) to evenly distribute pressure. Custom-made insoles often combine both approaches by layering soft top covers over rigid posting. Recently computer-aided design and manufacturing CAD/CAM technology has streamlined custom-made insole production; digital foot scans are processed by software, and insoles are milled or 3D printed from precise designs [4, 5]. Studies show CAD/CAM insoles can achieve even better pressure relief than traditional plaster-cast insoles. Quantitative statistical CAD/CAM design reduced high-pressure regions by an additional 15% compared to conventional total-contact insoles. 3D printed insoles are emerging approaches, enabling intricate porous structures tailored to the patient's arch and load pattern [6]. The choice of insole type should consider the patient's risk, foot anatomy, and resources, balancing offloading efficacy against cost and production time.

## 4.3 Insoles Material and Design Features

Effective insoles integrate several design elements to cushion the foot and redistribute plantar pressure. Materials play a crucial role in insole design—softer foams (EVA, urethane, Poron) deform under load to redistribute pressure, whereas rigid materials (cork, hard EVA) provide structural support. Biomechanical studies show that soft insole materials significantly outperform stiff materials in reducing peak plantar pressure [7]. Instead of using single material in insole fabrication, dual-layer or multilayer materials are frequently prescribed to achieve multifunction from a single insole [8, 9]. This includes a soft top layer to provide comfort and pressure relief, a middle layer for shock absorption, and a firmer base for arch and structural support and maintaining the correct alignment of foot. Firm and soft material supporting elements can be included depending on the foot complication. These elements include deep heel cups (to stabilize the calcaneus and limit pronation), contoured arch supports (to offload the midfoot), and metatarsal pads or bars (placed proximal to metatarsal heads). Accurate placement of metatarsal pads and additional features significantly reduced forefoot pressure [10]. In clinical practice, lateral heel wedges, and localized cutouts under bony prominences are commonly used to fine-tune pressure relief and enhance offloading efficacy.

Cushioning top layer is often used to protect high-risk areas; cushion materials have large cell sizes and absorb impact well. Multilayer constructions may include a combination of soft material as top cushioning property, shock absorption material as middle layer, and stiff material as base layer to maximize the offloading of abnormal peak plantar pressure. Insole design balances offloading performance, comfort, and durability; soft, breathable, and moisture wicking covers improve patient adherence, whereas firmer material ensures total contact fit without bottoming out.

## 4.4 Integration of Advanced Technologies in Insole Prescription

Recent advances offer novel ways to fabricate and personalize patient-specific insoles. CAD/CAM uses 3D foot scanning and modeling software to create precise foot orthosis. Research indicates CAD/CAM designed insoles can outperform traditional insoles: a study using a qualitative statistical CAD algorithm reduced high-pressure regions by approximately 15% more than traditionally fabricated insoles. This digital approach also shortens production time and reduces manual variability. Additive manufacturing (3D printing) is increasingly applied to fabricate insoles.

Fused deposition modeling (FDM) and selective laser sintering (SLS) allow the creation of complex internal structures (honeycombs, lattices, etc.) that provide targeted flexibility and cushioning. SLS can fabricate durable nylon insoles with variable porosity to relieve specific high-pressure areas. 3D printing supports rapid prototyping and individualization (multi-density or materials print), although concerns remain about material fatigue and print resolution [11].

Artificial intelligence (AI) and machine learning are opening new frontiers in insole design and customization. Deep-learning models have been developed to classify diabetic feet based on morphology and complications using 3D scans that can guide personalized insole strategies. A convolutional neural network achieved over 82% accuracy in categorizing diabetic foot arch types (flat, normal, cavus) directly from 3D foot images [12]. Such algorithms could eventually suggest optimal insole geometries or modifications for a given patient. Researchers are also investigating inverse design methods; given a desired pressure mapping, AI could compute the internal structure of an insole (varying lattice density) to achieve appropriate desire offloading.

Wearable sensor integration is another emerging trend for insole prescription. Insoles embedded with pressure sensors and connected to mobile devices can provide real-time feedback. A notable proof of concept trial showed that an intelligent insole system (with plantar pressure sensing and smart alerts) reduced ulcer recurrence by 71% compared to standard care [13]. Although preliminary, this suggests that feedback-driven offloading, alerting the patient to shift weight, can significantly improve outcomes. The integration of flexible sensors (temperature, moisture, and gait) into insoles is also being explored to create fully smart orthoses. These technologies hold promises for improving comfort, fitness, and offloading precision, but clinical adoption will require validation of long-term safety and cost-effectiveness.

## 4.5 Clinical Evaluation Tools and Outcome Measures

Clinical studies of diabetic insoles use a variety of primary and secondary outcome measures. The gold standard primary outcome in prevention trials is usually foot ulceration incidence. Standardized tools facilitate objective assessment of diabetic neuropathy and plantar pressure. In neuropathy, a 10-gram Semmes-Weinstein monofilament is the clinical benchmark as inability to feel this bulking filament at one or more plantar sites denotes loss of protective sensation. A 128-Hz tuning fork or biothesiometer can quantify vibration threshold. These simple sensory tests predict ulcer risk and guide interventions. Vascular assessments include Doppler-derived ankle-brachial index (ABI) and toe pressures. Palpating pedal pulses and measuring skin temperature with more than 2 °C difference can also reveal circulation issues or early Charcot changes. In biomechanical trials, primary outcomes often include quantitative pressure metrics: peak plantar pressure, contact areas, and pressure time integral [14, 15] (Fig. 4.3). Secondary outcomes encompass functional and patient-reported foot health and disability and diabetes-specific quality-of-life instruments. These assess pain, activity limitations, and emotional impact of

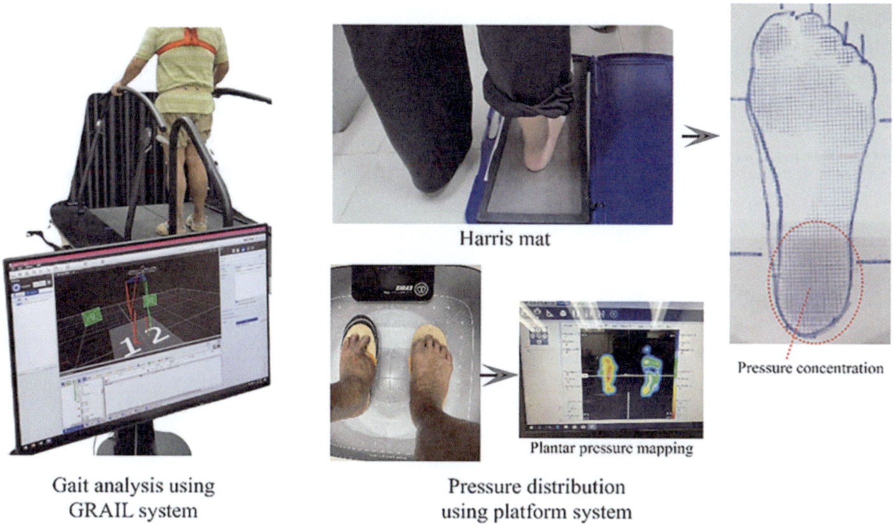


**Fig. 4.3** Outcome measurement tool to analyze kinetic and kinematic data and plantar pressure distribution

foot problems. Adherence to insole use (hours per day worn) and footwear satisfaction are also tracked, as noncompliance can dilute treatment effects. Other secondary end points may include callus area, gait parameters, or ulcer recurrence rate [13, 16].

Consistently measuring and reporting these outcomes is critical for research comparability. Pressure reduction and ulcer healing are the most widely used end points and has recommended a core outcome set for diabetic foot trials to standardize reporting. In practice, in-shoe pressure analysis (Tekscan F-scan or Novel Pedar system) is used to capture plantar pressure profiles during walking or other assigned activities, while clinical exam and photography document ulceration and history of complications. The threshold for clinically significant change remains an area of study, but in general substantial drop in peak plantar pressure often more than 20–30% is sought as evidence of effective offloading [17]. Plantar pressure measurement devices with a well-established threshold peak plantar pressure of 200 kPa (measure in-shoe) are a commonly cited threshold above which ulceration risk rises markedly [17, 18]. Moreover, most clinical protocols aim to keep pressure below this level by insole modification. A more practical benchmark comes from IWGDF guidelines; therapeutic footwear including insoles should achieve at least a 30% reduction in peak plantar pressure compared to standard shoes. Pressure mapping systems quantify these metrics and validate the effectiveness of offloading designs. Calibration and repeat testing are crucial, as factors like shoe fitness and walking speed can affect reading.

To reduce the risk factors, it is important to detect loss of sensation using monofilament and identify high-pressure areas using pressure sensors. An insole prescription is considered successful if follow-up measurements show substantial offloading of previously vulnerable areas. Custom-made insoles and prefabricated insoles can play a crucial role in managing various lower limb injuries including diabetic foot ulceration. Integration of advanced technologies in insole prescription has been introduced to increase precision and reduce time-consuming. The quantitative criteria with the baseline pressure less than 200 kPa to drop by at least 25–35% together with healing of existing lesions guide ongoing insole modification and patient management with a well-organized follow-up plan.

## References

1. Bus SA, Sacco ICN, Monteiro-Soares M, Raspovic A, Paton J, Rasmussen A, et al. Guidelines on the prevention of foot ulcers in persons with diabetes (IWGDF 2023 update). Diabetes Metab Res Rev. 2024;40(3):e3651.
2. Paton JS, Stenhouse EA, Bruce G, Zahra D, Jones RB. A comparison of customised and prefabricated insoles to reduce risk factors for neuropathic diabetic foot ulceration: a participant-blinded randomised controlled trial. J Foot Ankle Res. 2012;5(1):31.
3. Hellstrand Tang U, Zügner R, Lisovskaja V, Karlsson J, Hagberg K, Tranberg R. Comparison of plantar pressure in three types of insole given to patients with diabetes at risk of developing foot ulcers – a two-year, randomized trial. J Clin Transl Endocrinol. 2014;1(4):121–32.
4. Smith D, Burgess E. The use of CAD/CAM technology in prosthetics and orthotics – current clinical models and a view to the future. J Rehabil Res Dev. 2001;38:327–34.
5. Huang C-N, Lee M-Y, Chang CC. Computer-aided design and manufacturing of customized insoles. IEEE Comput Graph Appl. 2011;31:74–9.
6. Chatpun S, Dissaneewate T, Kwanyuang A, Nouman M, Srewaradachpisal S, Movrin D. Infill pattern and density of 3D-printed insoles Alter energy and pressure distribution in gait. Appl Sci [Internet]. 2025;15(7):3916.
7. Peng H-T, Liu L-W, Chen C-J, Chen Z-R. The soft prefabricated orthopedic insole decreases plantar pressure during uphill walking with heavy load carriage. Bioengineering [Internet]. 2023;10(3):353.
8. Nouman M, Chong DYR, Chatpun S. Finite element approach towards selection of appropriate materials to redistribute peak plantar pressure in diabetic foot with neuropathy: selecting appropriate materials for diabetic foot. PSU Med J. 2021;1(2):43–54.
9. Nouman M, Dissaneewate T, Leelasamran W, Chatpun S. The insole materials influence the plantar pressure distributions in diabetic foot with neuropathy during different walking activities. Gait Posture. 2019;74:154–61.
10. Lee PY, Landorf KB, Bonanno DR, Menz HB. Comparison of the pressure-relieving properties of various types of forefoot pads in older people with forefoot pain. J Foot Ankle Res. 2014;7(1):18.
11. Salles AS, Gyi DE. The specification of personalised insoles using additive manufacturing. Work (Reading, Mass). 2012;41(Suppl 1):1771–4.
12. Li PL, Xiao QF, Yick KL, Liu QL, Zhang LY. A novel deep learning approach to classify 3D foot types of diabetic patients. Sci Rep. 2025;15(1):13819.
13. Abbott C, Chatwin K, Foden P, Hasan A, Sange C, Rajbhandari S, et al. Innovative intelligent insole system reduces diabetic foot ulcer recurrence at plantar sites: a prospective, randomised, proof-of-concept study. Lancet Digit Health. 2019;1:e308–e18.
14. Ramadhan GT, Haris F, Jan Y-K, Liau B-Y, Chang W-T, Tai C-C, et al. Effect of different inner pressures of air insoles and walking durations on plantar pressure time integral. Sci Rep. 2024;14(1):19272.
15. Melai T, Ijzerman T, Schaper N, Lange T, Willems P, Meijer K, et al. Calculation of plantar pressure time integral, an alternative approach. Gait Posture. 2011;34:379–83.

16. Tedeschi R, Giorgi F, Donati D. Footwear and foot health: unveiling the role of proper shoe fit in preventing podiatric issues and enhancing well-being. Appl Sci [Internet]. 2024;14(21):9938.
17. Castro-Martins P, Marques A, Coelho L, Vaz M, Costa JT. Plantar pressure thresholds as a strategy to prevent diabetic foot ulcers: a systematic review. Heliyon. 2024;10(4):e26161.
18. D'Amico M, Kinel E, Roncoletta P, Gnaldi A, Ceppitelli C, Belli F, et al. Data-driven CAD-CAM vs traditional total contact custom insoles: a novel quantitative-statistical framework for the evaluation of insoles offloading performance in diabetic foot. PLoS One. 2021;16(3):e0247915.

# Gait Training and Exercise for Diabetics Foot Complications

5

Pannika Prachgosin and Tulaya Dissaneewate

## 5.1 Importance of Gait Training and Exercise in Managing Diabetic Foot Complications

Diabetic foot complications, including diabetic foot ulcer (DFU), Charcot neuroarthropathy, diabetic foot infections, and lower extremity amputations, contribute significantly to the global burden of disability [1, 2]. Diabetic peripheral neuropathy (DPN)—affecting motor, sensory, and autonomic systems—and ischemia are the key underlying pathologies of diabetic foot conditions [2]. Motor neuropathy leads to foot deformities and biomechanical abnormalities, such as increased plantar pressure. Sensory neuropathy results in the loss of protective sensations, including pain and temperature perception. Autonomic neuropathy causes decreased sweating, which leads to dry skin that is more prone to breakdown.

DFUs commonly develop due to repetitive loading on vulnerable areas of the foot. Peripheral artery disease (PAD) further exacerbates the issue by reducing blood flow, contributing to the formation of nonhealing ulcers. Patients with diabetes have a 19–34% annual risk of developing DFUs, with a recurrence rate of 40% within 1 year after ulcer healing [3, 4]. Factors contributing to DFU recurrence can be biological, behavioral, or a combination of both, including poor diabetes control, progression of DPN or PAD, and improper management of offloading devices. Unhealed ulcers can lead to lower limb amputation [5].

P. Prachgosin (✉)
Department of Rehabilitation Medicine, Faculty of Medicine Siriraj Hospital, Mahidol University, Bangkok, Thailand
e-mail: Pannika.prc@mahidol.ac.th

T. Dissaneewate
Department of Rehabilitation Medicine, Faculty of Medicine, Prince of Songkla University, Hat Yai, Songkhla, Thailand
tulaya.p@psu.ac.th



M. Nouman, S. Chatpun (eds.), *A Comprehensive Guide to Insole-Based Approaches for Diabetic Foot Complications*,
https://doi.org/10.1007/978-981-95-0656-9_5

To prevent foot ulcers in diabetic patients, the International Working Group on the Diabetic Foot (IWGDF) guideline in 2023 recommends walking with suitable foot protection, such as properly fitting, accommodating, and therapeutic footwear, especially for individuals at moderate to high risk, and monitoring foot skin temperature [6]. Additionally, the IWGDF 2023 suggests that foot-related exercises and increasing daily weight-bearing walking activity by an extra 1000 steps per day with appropriate footwear are likely to be safe for patients at low-to-moderate risk of ulceration.

Lower limb exercises can improve circulation, enhance nerve function, increase muscle strength and flexibility, improve gait, and reduce the risk of complications [7, 8]. These exercises include ankle mobility drills, sensorimotor training, lower limb strengthening, balance exercises, and gait training, with a focus on low-impact activities. The immediate effects of an 8-week sensorimotor and gait training program, as demonstrated in Ahmad I. and colleagues' study, showed significant improvements in nerve function through increased nerve conduction velocity. Muscle function related to postural control at the ankle and trunk levels improved, as evidenced by reduced electromyography (EMG) activities of the tibialis anterior (TA) and medial gastrocnemius (MG) muscles and a decreased angle of mini board difference during standing balance evaluation. Walking improvements were observed through increased EMG activities of the TA and MG muscles, which likely enhanced shock absorption and push-off power, while reduced multifidus activity helped minimize trunk forward compensation [9]. In a one-year study by Monteiro RL and colleagues, a 12-week foot exercise program also successfully maintained fast gait speed and vibration perception, further supporting the role of targeted exercises in managing diabetic foot complications [10].

## 5.2 Types of Exercise for Diabetic Foot Complications

Most diabetic patients are physically inactive or lead a sedentary lifestyle. Physical inactivity is one of the modifiable risk factors for developing diabetic macrovascular and microvascular complications, which are the main causes of morbidity and mortality [11]. In addition to lifestyle modification, dietary control, and medication, exercise therapy is an intervention that should be recommended to diabetic patients. Exercise therapy has been shown to reduce the incidence of cardiovascular events, microvascular complications, and all-cause mortality in individuals with diabetes [11].

Recent evidence suggests that physical activity and exercise therapy may improve outcomes related to diabetic foot complications [7, 12]. Exercise therapy has positively influenced pathological factors associated with DPN by promoting microvascular function and fat oxidation, reducing oxidative stress, and increasing neurotrophic factors, which collectively contribute to a reduced risk of neuropathy development in diabetic patients [7].

### 5.2.1 General Exercise Recommendations

According to many international guidelines for diabetes management such as the European Society of Cardiology, the American College of Sports Medicine, and the American Diabetes Association, exercise therapy recommendations include aerobic, resistance, flexibility, and balance exercises [13–15]. These guidelines advise engaging in 150–300 min of moderate-intensity aerobic physical activity or 75–150 min of vigorous-intensity aerobic physical activity per week, in addition to moderate-intensity resistance exercises (50–69% of one repetition maximum, 10–15 repetitions per set, 1–3 sets per type of exercise) two or more times per week on nonconsecutive days for adults with diabetes. During exercise therapy programs, diabetic patients should protect their feet by avoiding walking barefoot and should wear properly fitting footwear.

In patients with diabetic foot complications, there is a common concern regarding exercise-induced foot ulceration or skin breakdown due to repetitive pressure on the plantar surface of the foot, particularly in patients with DPN who have impaired protective sensation. Recent research has demonstrated that physical activity can reduce the risk of skin breakdown, and weight-bearing exercise does not increase the risk of foot ulceration if prescribed appropriately [16]. Nevertheless, exercise therapy programs should be carefully tailored for patients with advanced foot deformities or active foot ulcerations.

To mitigate the risk of foot ulceration and skin breakdown, every diabetic patient should undergo a foot examination prior to the prescription of an exercise therapy program to determine if the patient is classified as foot-at-risk [6]. The IWGDF has stratified diabetic patients into four risk categories [6, 17]:

Risk category 0 (very low): Diabetic patient with no LOPS and no signs of PAD
Risk category 1 (low): Diabetic patient with LOPS or PAD
Risk category 2 (moderate): Diabetic patient with LOPS and PAD or LOPS with foot deformity or PAD with foot deformity
Risk category 3 (high): Diabetic patient with LOPS or PAD and one or more of history of foot ulcer, a lower extremity amputation (minor or major), and end-stage renal disease

A patient is considered foot-at-risk if they fall into IWGDF risk categories 1, 2, or 3.

#### 5.2.1.1 Exercise Recommendations for Foot-at-Risk with No Active Foot Ulceration

Studies involving patients classified under IWGDF risk categories 1–2 with DPN have shown that prescribing moderate-intensity weight-bearing exercise can improve walking distance without increasing the risk of foot ulceration [18, 19]. To reduce the risk of foot ulceration, individuals in the IWGDF foot-at-risk should gradually increase weight-bearing walking activity, limiting the increase to no more than 10% of total steps every 2 weeks [20]. It is important to ensure that patients wear appropriate footwear during their exercise program, gradually increasing the intensity of the exercises and frequently monitor their skin for pre-ulcerative signs or skin breakdown.

For patients with vasculopathy and claudication, an intermittent walking exercise program with a total duration exceeding 30 min per day for 3 days a week can significantly enhance walking speed and distance [21]. However, it is essential that the claudication score does not exceed 3 out of 4 during the exercise program.

Diabetic patients identified as foot-at-risk without active foot ulceration should be encouraged to engage in weight-bearing exercises rather than non-weight-bearing exercises [18, 19]. Furthermore, combining an aerobic exercise program with lower extremity muscle strengthening and balance training has the potential to reduce the long-term incidence rate of foot lesions by 44.6% [7].

#### 5.2.1.2 Exercise Recommendations for Foot-at-Risk with Active Foot Ulceration

Patients with diabetes who have active foot ulcers should refrain from weight-bearing exercises to minimize pressure on the ulcerated area. While the evidence supporting exercise as an intervention to promote the healing of DFUs remains limited, non-weight-bearing exercise programs may offer potential benefits [22, 23]. Therefore, such exercise regimens should be recommended for patients with DFUs, provided they are designed by healthcare professionals. Additionally, patients should be closely monitored throughout the course of the exercise program to ensure safe and effective management of their condition. Some examples of weight-bearing and non-weight-bearing exercise for diabetic foot patients are illustrated in Fig. 5.1.

### 5.2.2 Foot-Related Exercise for Diabetic Foot Complications

In patients with foot-at-risk, DPN causes impaired sensation and proprioception in the lower extremities, muscle weakness in the foot and ankle, and reduced mobility in the foot and ankle joints. Additionally, elevated blood glucose levels can lead to collagen tissue stiffness, which further contributes to joint rigidity. These combined factors reduce the range of motion in the foot and ankle joints, promote structural foot deformities, impair balance, and alter gait (e.g., shortened step length, wide-based gait pattern, and increased energy expenditure during walking) [24]. Furthermore, abnormal plantar pressure, particularly in the forefoot and midfoot during the gait cycle, increases the risk of foot ulceration and enhances susceptibility to falls [24].

Foot-related exercises, which include foot-ankle exercises and balance and gait training, are recommended for patients with foot-at-risk [6]. These exercises aim to address modifiable risk factors for foot ulceration, as previously outlined.

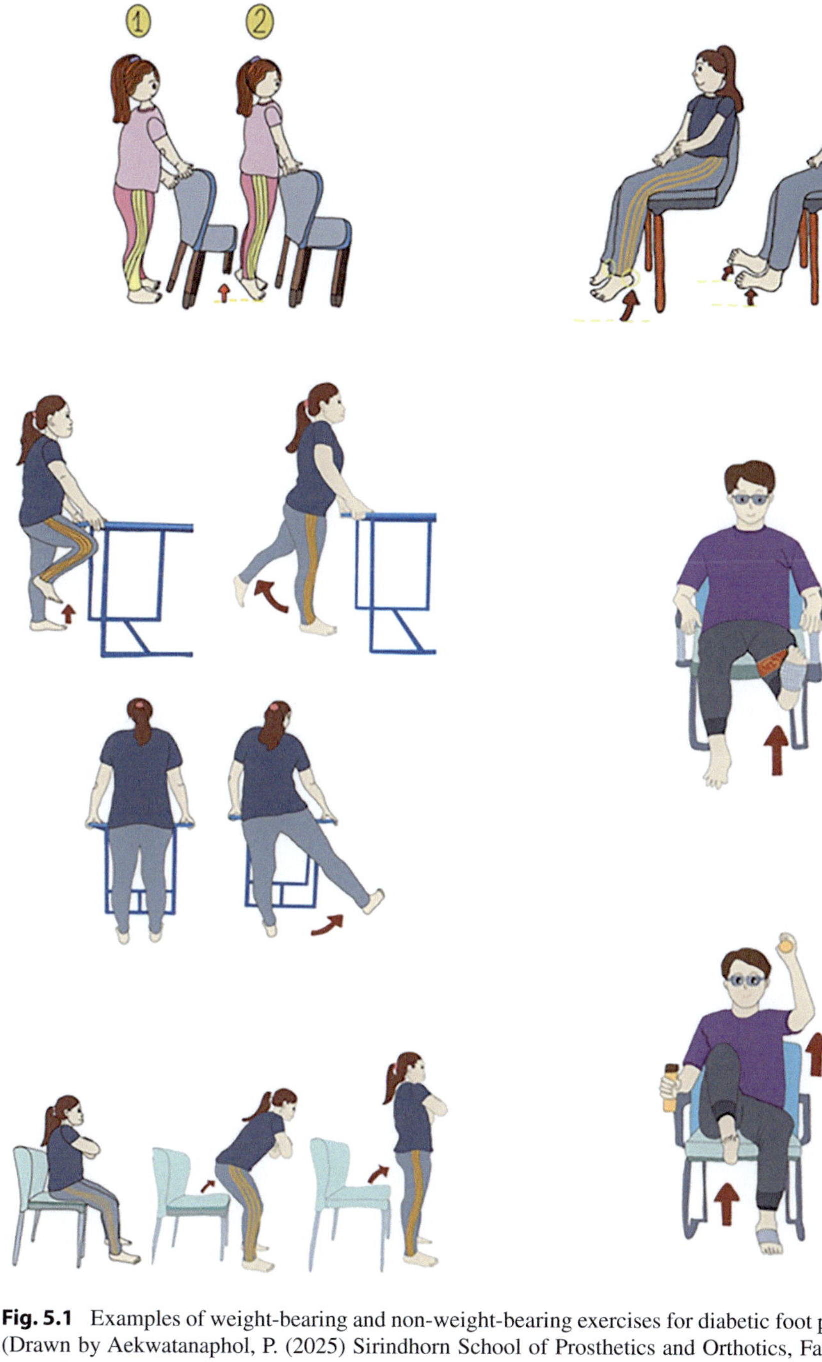


**Fig. 5.1** Examples of weight-bearing and non-weight-bearing exercises for diabetic foot patients. (Drawn by Aekwatanaphol, P. (2025) Sirindhorn School of Prosthetics and Orthotics, Faculty of Medicine, Siriraj Hospital, Mahidol University, Bangkok)

#### 5.2.2.1 Foot-Ankle Exercise

Foot-ankle exercises offer several benefits, including improvements in the range of motion of the foot and ankle joints, alleviation of neuropathic signs and symptoms, and more balanced plantar pressure distribution. Range of motion exercises should be applied to all joints within the foot and ankle (see Fig. 5.2) and can be performed either actively or passively by the patient. Research indicates that the range of motion in these joints can improve significantly after 5 weeks of consistent joint mobilization [25, 26]. Additionally, stretching and strengthening the muscles of the lower legs can help alleviate tension in plantar flexion, thereby reducing forefoot plantar pressure during the gait cycle [18, 25, 26] (see Fig. 5.3).

In diabetic patients with pre-ulcerative lesions, IWGDF risk category 3, or those with active foot ulcers, foot-related exercise should be performed in a seated position. In other cases, these exercises may be conducted in a standing or weight-bearing position, if tolerated [6].

#### 5.2.2.2 Balance and Gait Training Exercise

In foot-at-risk patients with DPN, the combination of decreased sensation and proprioception in the lower extremities, along with reduced range of motion in the foot and ankle joints, can lead to postural instability, gait abnormalities, and abnormal plantar pressure during the gait cycle [24]. As a result, these individuals are at an increased risk of falling. Balance and gait training exercises should be prescribed to improve postural control and coordination during walking or dynamic activities, which can help reduce the risk of falls and alleviate the fear of falling. Various balance and gait training programs are available, and patients should be guided to select a program appropriate for their balance and coordination abilities (see Fig. 5.4). Additionally, these exercises should be performed in a protective and safe environment.

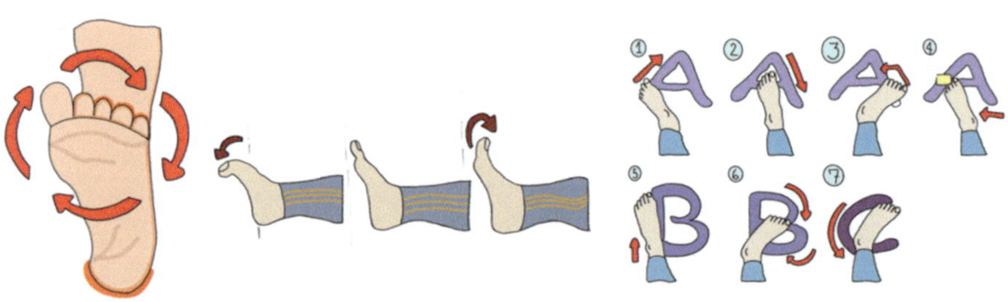

**Fig. 5.2** Example of the foot-ankle exercise; range of motion exercise of the foot and ankle. (Drawn by Aekwatanaphol, P. (2025) Sirindhorn School of Prosthetics and Orthotics, Faculty of Medicine, Siriraj Hospital, Mahidol University, Bangkok)

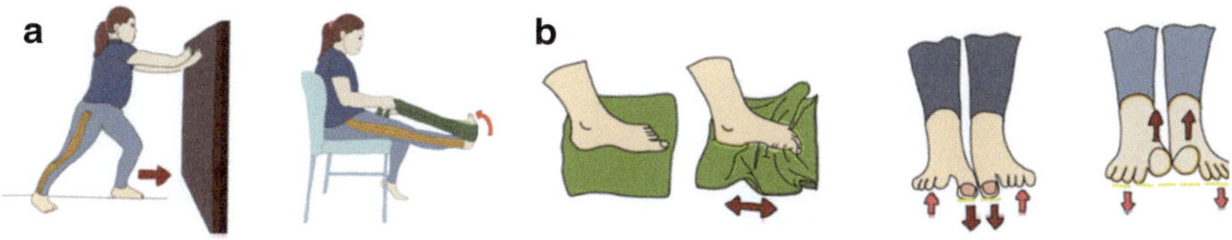


**Fig. 5.3** Example of the foot-ankle exercise. (**a**) Stretching exercise of lower leg muscles; gastrocnemius-soleus and hamstring muscles. (**b**) Strengthening exercise of intrinsic foot muscles. (Drawn by Aekwatanaphol, P. (2025) Sirindhorn School of Prosthetics and Orthotics, Faculty of Medicine, Siriraj Hospital, Mahidol University, Bangkok)

### 5.2.3 Special Consideration in Exercise Therapy Program

Exercise therapy programs for foot-at-risk diabetic patients can be implemented either as home-based or hospital-based programs. However, studies have shown that exercise programs conducted in a supervised setting over 8–12 weeks—whether face-to-face or via telemedicine and either individually or in groups—can enhance motivation through feedback [6, 18]. In these settings, the therapists can encourage patients to meet the minimum required exercise dose, which may increase the likelihood of patients continuing their exercise regimen after the program concludes, thereby promoting a healthier lifestyle and behavior.

Additionally, every diabetic patient prescribed an exercise program should receive education on the importance of wearing appropriate footwear, regularly monitoring their feet for skin lesions or breakdowns, and recognizing any abnormal symptoms during exercise, such as signs of cardiovascular events, hypoglycemia, or musculoskeletal pain and soreness.

## 5.3 Integration of Insoles with Gait Training and Exercise

During gait training and exercise, patients experience increased plantar loading and shearing forces, which contributes to elevated plantar pressure and temperature, potentially leading to DFUs. The degree of pressure and temperature change depends on the type of activity and walking speed [27]. Therefore, insoles play a crucial role in gait training and exercise for diabetic patients by reducing plantar pressure. Additionally, insoles may enhance sensory feedback, regulate muscle activity and balance control, and provide monitoring feedback to identify ulceration risks [28–33].

According to the IWGDF guidelines, proper footwear and offloading devices, such as customized insoles, should be considered for patients with DPN during weight-bearing activities in daily life, particularly for those at moderate to high risk of ulcers [6]. A systematic review found that customized insoles significantly reduced peak plantar pressure (PP) both immediately and in the long term when patients adhered to wearing footwear for at least 4 h per day [31]. Muller K and colleagues reported that the peak forefoot PP for patients with DPN who walked 2844–4972 strides per day ranged from 23.6 to 37.8 $N/cm^2$, with a daily cumulative

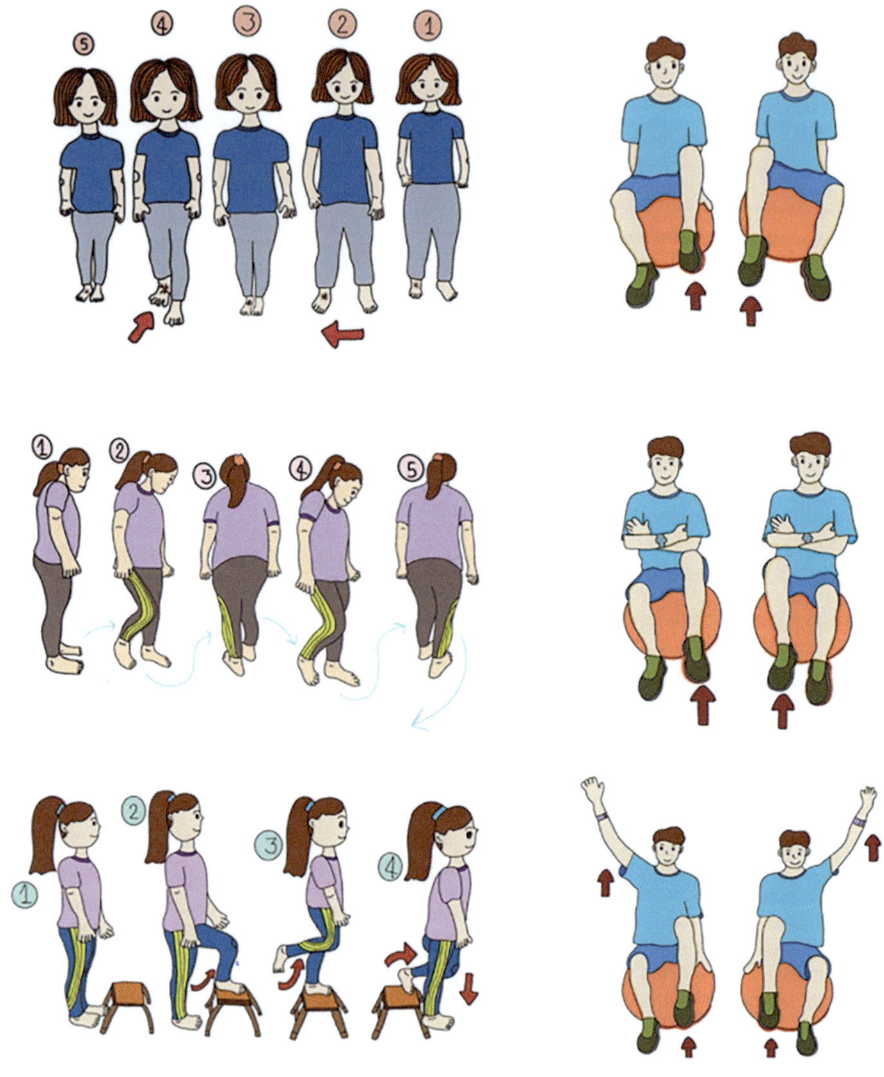

**Fig. 5.4** Example of balance and gait training exercise in weight-bearing and non-weight-bearing positions. (Drawn by Aekwatanaphol, P. (2025) Sirindhorn School of Prosthetics and Orthotics, Faculty of Medicine, Siriraj Hospital, Mahidol University, Bangkok)

forefoot stress of 248.35–459.68 MPa·s/day [34]. Currently, there is no consensus on the optimal cumulative plantar tissue loading required to prevent DFUs. Despite this, the optimal physical activity intensity for individuals with diabetes that does not increase DFU risk remains unclear and controversial [35].

The design and cover materials of customized insoles also influence sensory perception and neuromuscular control and balance in patients with DPN [33, 36, 37]. Center of pressure (COP) velocity is one of the biomechanical parameters that reflects fall risk, with lower COP velocity during standing indicating better balance [38]. Previous studies have reported conflicting results regarding insole firmness, arch support, and cup design, as these factors may have either positive or negative effects on COP parameters. The variability in outcomes may be due to differences in neuropathy severity among study participants. To confirm the balance-related effects of insoles, longitudinal studies are needed.

In the era of emerging technology, customized insoles for patients with DPN have been enhanced with assistive features to improve foot function. For example, since individuals with DPN experience sensory deficits, sensory enhancement is considered a promising strategy for gait training [39]. Vibrating shoe insoles have been proposed to amplify sensation in insensate feet, thereby improving neuromuscular control and balance [30, 40]. Orlando and colleagues found that patients with DPN exhibited reduced ankle plantar flexor activation and decreased COP velocity while using insoles with vibrational stimuli while quiet standing with eyes closed [40]. However, the results from these studies were based on small sample sizes and showed only immediate effects. Further research is needed to evaluate the long-term effectiveness of such intervention.

Besides plantar pressure, temperature at the plantar surface is considered a surrogate measure for shear stress. According to the IWGDF recommendations, temperature should be monitored during daily activities. If the temperature difference between corresponding regions of the left and right foot exceeds a threshold of 2.2 °C (or 4.0 °F) on two consecutive days, it is a sign of impending ulceration [6, 41]. Temperature and Pressure Monitoring and Regulating Insoles (TAPMARI) is a multilayer insole equipped with a cooling system housed in an enclosure attached to the subject's calf [42]. A study by Yavuz and colleagues demonstrated the effectiveness of TAPMARI in regulating temperature below the soft tissue injury threshold (less than 35 °C) during a two-hour walking session, while also maintaining a relatively even pressure distribution, with PP below 200 kPa. However, the temperature target in this study did not focus on the temperature difference as suggested by the IWGDF guidelines. Further research is needed to confirm the long-term effects of temperature-regulating insoles on DFU prevention.

Ideally, diabetic footwear and offloading devices should be integrated into exercise and gait training programs to reduce ulceration risk and enhance training effectiveness. However, without a monitoring sensor system, customized insoles are unable to measure cumulative plantar loading or temperature changes, nor can they provide real-time feedback to optimize exercise training outcomes.

## 5.4 Role of AI in Gait Analysis and Training

A monitoring and biofeedback system that measures plantar pressure and temperature is an effective method for improving locomotion and reducing the risk of DFUs in patients with diabetes [27, 43, 44]. This system relies on artificial intelligence (AI) for continuous data collection, processing, and pattern recognition of physiological responses that may indicate an increased risk of falling or ulceration. Additionally, it provides real-time feedback to help mitigate these risks.

Currently, the system has been developed to incorporate force/pressure sensors and gyroscopes with features such as lightweight design, reduced bulk, increased flexibility, and self-rechargeability. However, force and pressure sensors still have limitations, including durability concerns, relatively high-power consumption, and low robustness. These sensors primarily evaluate vertical force, making it difficult to assess shear forces, which also contribute to DFU development. These limitations may restrict the long-term usability of force and pressure sensors in daily life for patients with DPN. At present, only one smart insole system has been studied in relation to DFU risk monitoring during activities: the SurroSense Rx (Orpyx Medical Technologies Inc., Calgary, AB, Canada) [42, 45–47].

The SurroSense Rx is an intelligent insole system equipped with eight plantar sensors, each measuring 0.6 mm in thickness, with a sampling rate of 8 Hz to monitor low sustained plantar pressure during daily activities. The device provides audiovisual and vibrational alerts on a smartwatch to notify patients of high integrated pressure, encouraging them to offload pressure accordingly. However, a systematic review has found no consensus on the cut-off threshold for plantar pressure associated with ulceration risk [48]. While most studies and the IWGDF guidelines recommend that customized offloading devices should aim for a peak plantar pressure reduction of less than 30% or below 200 kPa, the alarm threshold used in the SurroSense Rx differs from those in most studies [47]. A study by Abbott and colleagues suggested that prolonged loading on plantar tissue, such as standing for more than 15 min, can impair capillary blood flow. The study hypothesized a low-pressure threshold of 35 mmHg as a critical value for daily activities [47, 48]. The SurroSense Rx system categorizes pressure levels based on exceeding capillary pressure (≥35 mmHg for 15 min) into three risk levels:

- High risk (95–100% of readings ≥35 mmHg)
- Moderate risk (35–94% of readings ≥35 mmHg)
- Low risk (0–34% of readings ≥35 mmHg)

An 18-month study of the SurroSense Rx in patients with moderate-to-severe DPN found a reduction in the number of bouts of high-pressure exposure after more than 16 weeks of wearing the device [32]. However, further research is needed to determine whether peak plantar pressure or low sustained pressure during weight-bearing activities plays a more significant role in ulceration risk.

## 5.5 Conclusion

Gait training and exercise are important for patients with diabetes to improve neuromuscular and enhance peripheral blood flow. The risk of DFU is increased due to increased plantar loading and shearing force during exercise training. Together with customized insoles and smart insoles system, patients can increase physical fitness with less risk of DFU. However, smart insoles system and further study are still needed to develop to improve exercise training effectiveness in patients with diabetes.

## References


1. Zhang Y, Lazzarini PA, McPhail SM, van Netten JJ, Armstrong DG, Pacella RE. Global disability burdens of diabetes-related lower-extremity complications in 1990 and 2016. Diabetes Care. 2020;43:964–74.
2. Edmonds M, Manu C, Vas P. The current burden of diabetic foot disease. J Clin Orthop Trauma. 2021;17:88–93.
3. Armstrong DG, Boulton AJM, Bus SA. Diabetic foot ulcers and their recurrence. N Engl J Med. 2017;376:2367–75.
4. Dubský M, Jirkovská A, Bem R, Fejfarová V, Skibová J, Schaper NC, et al. Risk factors for recurrence of diabetic foot ulcers: prospective follow-up analysis in the Eurodiale subgroup. Int Wound J. 2013;10:555–61.
5. Pecoraro RE, Reiber GE, Burgess EM. Pathways to diabetic limb amputation: basis for prevention. Diabetes Care. 1990;13:513–21.
6. Bus SA, Sacco ICN, Monteiro-Soares M, Raspovic A, Paton J, Rasmussen A, et al. Guidelines on the prevention of foot ulcers in persons with diabetes (IWGDF 2023 update). Diabetes Metab Res Rev. 2024:40.
7. Matos M, Mendes R, Silva AB, Sousa N. Physical activity and exercise on diabetic foot related outcomes: a systematic review. Diabetes Res Clin Pract. 2018;139:81–90.
8. Aydin E, Ertuğrul MB. The role of rehabilitation in the management of diabetic foot wounds. Turk J Phys Med Rehabil. 2021;67:389–98.
9. Ahmad I, Verma S, Noohu MM, Shareef MY, Ejaz HM. Sensorimotor and gait training improves proprioception, nerve function, and muscular activation in patients with diabetic peripheral neuropathy: a randomized control trial. J Musculoskelet Neuronal Interact. 2020;20:234.
10. Monteiro RL, Ferreira JSSP, Silva ÉQ, Cruvinel-Júnior RH, Veríssimo JL, Bus SA, et al. Foot–ankle therapeutic exercise program can improve gait speed in people with diabetic neuropathy: a randomized controlled trial. Sci Rep. 2022;12:1–12.
11. Rietz M, Lehr A, Mino E, Lang A, Szczerba E, Schiemann T, et al. Physical activity and risk of major diabetes-related complications in individuals with diabetes: a systematic review and meta-analysis of observational studies. Diabetes Care. 2022;45:3101–11.
12. Francia P, Gulisano M, Anichini R, Seghieri G. Diabetic foot and exercise therapy: step by step the role of rigid posture and biomechanics treatment. Curr Diabetes Rev. 2014;10:86–99.
13. Bull FC, Al-Ansari SS, Biddle S, Borodulin K, Buman MP, Cardon G, et al. World Health Organization 2020 guidelines on physical activity and sedentary behaviour. Br J Sports Med. 2020;54:1451.
14. Kanaley JA, Colberg SR, Corcoran MH, Malin SK, Rodriguez NR, Crespo CJ, et al. Exercise/physical activity in individuals with type 2 diabetes: a consensus statement from the American College of Sports Medicine. Med Sci Sports Exerc. 2022;54:353–68.
15. Committee ADAPP, ElSayed NA, Aleppo G, Bannuru RR, Beverly EA, Bruemmer D, et al. Summary of revisions: standards of care in diabetes—2024. Diabetes Care. 2024;47:S5–10.
16. van Netten JJ, Fijen VM, Bus SA. Weight-bearing physical activity in people with diabetes-related foot disease: a systematic review. Diabetes Metab Res Rev. 2022;38:e3552.
17. Monteiro-Soares M, Hamilton EJ, Russell DA, Srisawasdi G, Boyko EJ, Mills JL, et al. Guidelines on the classification of foot ulcers in people with diabetes (IWGDF 2023 update). Diabetes Metab Res Rev. 2024;40:e3648.

18. van Netten JJ, Sacco ICN, Lavery L, Monteiro-Soares M, Paton J, Rasmussen A, et al. Clinical and biomechanical effectiveness of foot-ankle exercise programs and weight-bearing activity in people with diabetes and neuropathy: a systematic review and meta-analysis. Diabetes Metab Res Rev. 2024;40:e3649.
19. LeMaster JW, Mueller MJ, Reiber GE, Mehr DR, Madsen RW, Conn VS. Effect of weight-bearing activity on foot ulcer incidence in people with diabetic peripheral neuropathy: Feet first randomized controlled trial. Phys Ther. 2008;88:1385.
20. Fernando ME, Woelfel SL, Perry D, Najafi B, Khan T, Dubourdieu C, et al. Dosing activity and return to preulcer function in diabetes-related foot ulcer remission. J Am Podiatr Med Assoc. 2021;111
21. Treat-Jacobson D, McDermott MM, Bronas UG, Campia U, Collins TC, Criqui MH, et al. Optimal exercise programs for patients with peripheral artery disease: a scientific statement from the American Heart Association. Circulation. 2019;139:E10–33.
22. Tran MM, Haley MN. Does exercise improve healing of diabetic foot ulcers? A systematic review. J Foot Ankle Res. 2021;14(1):19.
23. Eraydin S, Avsar G. The effect of foot exercises on wound healing in type 2 diabetic patients with a foot ulcer: a randomized control study. J Wound Ostomy Continence Nurs. 2018;45:123–30.
24. Bursać SN, Talić G, Tomić N. The correlation between biomechanical parameters of lower limb and overall risk for diabetic foot ulcer. Scr Med (Brno). 2023;54:219–28.
25. Lepesis V, Paton J, Rickard A, Latour JM, Marsden J. Effects of foot and ankle mobilisations combined with home stretches in people with diabetic peripheral neuropathy: a proof-of-concept RCT. J Foot Ankle Res. 2023;16:88.
26. Cruvinel-Júnior RH, Ferreira JSSP, Veríssimo JL, Monteiro RL, Suda EY, Silva ÉQ, et al. Could an internet-based foot-ankle therapeutic exercise program modify clinical outcomes and gait biomechanics in people with diabetic neuropathy? A clinical proof-of-concept study. Sensors (Basel). 2022;22:9582.
27. Rosell-Diago MP, Izquierdo-Renau M, Julian-Rochina I, Arrébola M, Miralles M. Thermography, temperature, pressure force distribution and physical activity in diabetic foot: a systematic review. Appl Sci. 2024;14:8726.
28. Spolaor F, Guiotto A, Ciniglio A, Sawacha Z. The effect of custom insoles on muscle activity in diabetic individuals with neuropathy. Appl Sci (Switzerland). 2023;13:2326.
29. Hazari A, Maiya AG, Shivashankara KN. Foot kinetic and kinematic profile in type 2 diabetes mellitus with peripheral neuropathy: a hospital-based study from South India. J Am Podiatr Med Assoc. 2019;109:36–49.
30. Hatton AL, Chatfield MD, Cattagni T, Vicenzino B. The effects of vibrating shoe insoles on standing balance, walking, and ankle-foot muscle activity in adults with diabetic peripheral neuropathy. Gait Posture. 2024;111:8–13.
31. Korada H, Maiya A, Rao SK, Hande M. Effectiveness of customized insoles on maximum plantar pressure in diabetic foot syndrome: A systematic review. Diabetes Metab Syndr. 2020;14:1093–9.
32. Chatwin KE, Abbott CA, Rajbhandari SM, Reddy PN, Bowling FL, Boulton AJM, et al. An intelligent insole system with personalised digital feedback reduces foot pressures during daily life: an 18-month randomised controlled trial. Diabetes Res Clin Pract. 2021;181:109091.
33. Paton J, Glasser S, Collings R, Marsden J. Getting the right balance: insole design alters the static balance of people with diabetes and neuropathy. J Foot Ankle Res. 2016;9:1–11.
34. Maluf KS, Mueller MJ. Comparison of physical activity and cumulative plantar tissue stress among subjects with and without diabetes mellitus and a history of recurrent plantar ulcers. Clin Biomech. 2003;18:567–75.
35. Lung CW, Wu FL, Liao F, Pu F, Fan Y, Jan YK. Emerging technologies for the prevention and management of diabetic foot ulcers. J Tissue Viability. 2020;29:61–8.
36. Hatton AL, Chatfield MD, Gane EM, Maharaj JN, Cattagni T, Burns J, et al. The effects of wearing textured versus smooth shoe insoles for 4-weeks in people with diabetic peripheral neuropathy: a randomised controlled trial. Disabil Rehabil. 2024;47:751–61.

37. Horstink KA, van der Woude LHV, Hijmans JM. Effects of offloading devices on static and dynamic balance in patients with diabetic peripheral neuropathy: a systematic review. Rev Endocr Metab Disord. 2021;22:325–35.
38. Quijoux F, Nicolaï A, Chairi I, Bargiotas I, Ricard D, Yelnik A, et al. A review of center of pressure (COP) variables to quantify standing balance in elderly people: algorithms and open-access code*. Physiol Rep. American Physiological Society; 2021.9(22):e15067
39. Giri HS, Borkar P. Effects of sensory stimulation on balance and postural control in diabetic neuropathy: systematic review. Int J Res Med Sci. 2021;9:2090.
40. Orlando G, Brown S, Jude E, Bowling FL, Boulton AJM, Reeves ND. Acute effects of vibrating insoles on dynamic balance and gait quality in individuals with diabetic peripheral neuropathy: a randomized crossover study. Diabetes Care. 2024;47:1004–11.
41. Wijlens AM, Holloway S, Bus SA, van Netten JJ. An explorative study on the validity of various definitions of a 2·2°C temperature threshold as warning signal for impending diabetic foot ulceration. Int Wound J. 2017;14:1346–51.
42. Yavuz M, Ersen A, Monga A, Lavery LA, Garrett AG, Salem Y, et al. Temperature- and pressure-regulating insoles for prevention of diabetic foot ulcers. J Foot Ankle Surg. 2020;59:685–8.
43. De León RD, Allet L, Golay A, Philippe J, Assal JP, Hauert CA, et al. Biofeedback can reduce foot pressure to a safe level and without causing new at-risk zones in patients with diabetes and peripheral neuropathy. Diabetes Metab Res Rev. 2013;29:139–44.
44. Bus SA. Innovations in plantar pressure and foot temperature measurements in diabetes. Diabetes Metab Res Rev. 2016;32:221–6.
45. Almuteb I, Hua R, Wang Y. Smart insoles review (2008-2021): applications, potentials, and future. Smart Health Elsevier. 2022;25:100301.
46. Subramaniam S, Majumder S, Faisal AI, Jamal DM. Insole-based systems for health monitoring: current solutions and research challenges. Sensors (Multidisciplinary Digital Publishing Institute). 2022;22:438.
47. Abbott CA, Chatwin KE, Foden P, Hasan AN, Sange C, Rajbhandari SM, et al. Innovative intelligent insole system reduces diabetic foot ulcer recurrence at plantar sites: a prospective, randomised, proof-of-concept study. Lancet Digit Health. 2019;1:e308–18.
48. Castro-Martins P, Marques A, Coelho L, Vaz M, Costa JT. Plantar pressure thresholds as a strategy to prevent diabetic foot ulcers: a systematic review. Heliyon. 2024;10:e26161.

# Footwear for Diabetic Foot Complications

**6**

Muhammad Nouman

## 6.1 Shoe Design Philosophy and Biomechanical Principles

Therapeutic footwear for diabetic patients is engineered as a biomechanical intervention, addressing neuropathy, ischemia, and deformities. Key principles include plantar pressure redistribution, shock absorption, and tissue protection. Each component of the diabetic shoes from the outsole to the upper must harmonize with foot anatomy to mitigate abnormal plantar pressure and ulcer risk. Beyond general load management, each anatomical component of diabetic shoes plays a critical role. The toe box is the front part of the shoes that cover and protect the toes. Diabetic shoes feature a roomy, extra-depth toe box that matches the shape of the toes (including any deformities) so that no excessive pressure or friction occurs on the dorsal or tip surfaces of the toes. A high and wide toe box accommodates hammer toes, bunions, or dressings and prevents the formation of blisters or ulcers on the toes. The material is often soft or stretchable in this area, allowing movement during contact reducing the risk of interdigital friction and dorsal ulceration. The heel counter should offer firm support to stabilize the rearfoot, especially beneficial in patients with a valgus or varus heel deformity. A well-reinforced heel cup also enhances overall foot alignment during stance and terminal phases of the gait.

The insole system is a key interface between feet and shoes, providing cushioning and total contact support to redistribute plantar pressure away from bony prominences. Diabetic insoles are typically made of multilayers of materials like plastazote, polyurethane, EVA, and Poron that absorb shock and reduce peak pressure designed based on plantar pressure mapping, providing targeted offloading.

M. Nouman (✉)
Sirindhorn School of Prosthetics and Orthotics, Faculty of Medicine, Siriraj Hospital, Mahidol University, Bangkok, Thailand
e-mail: muhammad.nou@mahidol.ac.th



M. Nouman, S. Chatpun (eds.), *A Comprehensive Guide to Insole-Based Approaches for Diabetic Foot Complications*,
https://doi.org/10.1007/978-981-95-0656-9_6

Some designs incorporate metatarsal pads, heel cups, or medial arch supports tailored to the individual foot morphology. Midsole materials contribute to shock absorption; dual-density foams are often used to buffer ground reaction forces while maintaining postural control. The outsole design, especially the incorporation of a rocker profile, reduces dorsiflexion demands at the metatarsophalangeal joints. This is crucial for forefoot ulcer prevention. The position and radius of the rocker apex should align with the individual's high-pressure zones. Improper rocker design, however, can compromise balance and gait efficiency, highlighting the need for precise fabrication. Upper materials should be soft, breathable, and stretchable, commonly made from multi-density leather or synthetic mesh, with a seamless lining to prevent friction blisters or pressure points. Closures such as Velcro straps or elastic lacing systems facilitate secure fitting while allowing volume adjustment for swelling or dressings. The shank, a stiff reinforcement between the heel and ball of the foot, enhances torsional rigidity and redistributes pressure from vulnerable midfoot areas. It also improves the mechanical leverage of the rocker sole.

## 6.2 Biomechanical Rationale for Footwear in Diabetic Foot Management

Understanding how inclusion of stabilizers, rocker bottom soles, and cushioning materials integrate biomechanically allows clinicians to prescribe or modify footwear that not only fits but also functions as a therapeutic device. When thoughtfully combined, shoe anatomy supports natural gait, accommodates deformities, reduces plantar pressure, and helps maintain tissue integrity across varying stages of diabetic foot risk. Diabetic neuropathy and ischemia alter normal gait mechanics and foot structure, leading to abnormal load distribution, repetitive pressure, and shear stress; especially at the forefoot, areas with bony prominences and heel. Studies show that plantar pressure is highest under the forefoot during ambulation, where peak vertical forces can reach up to 120% of the body weight [1]. Properly designed diabetic footwear plays a critical role in redistributing plantar pressure especially under metatarsal heads, reducting shear and compressive forces, enhancing shock absorption to mitigate cumulative tissue trauma, accommodating deformities and rigid structures and offering protection against external mechanical and environmental trauma (Fig. 6.1).

## 6.3 Essential Design Features of Therapeutic Shoes

Footwear must be tailored to risk classification according to well-known foot care guidelines. There are certain key shoe features for diabetic foot that need to be considered. A critical design element includes a wide and deep toe box to accommodate foot deformities and prevent pressure points, paired with sufficient insole depth to house an insole without causing compression. Heel height is restricted to less than 2 cm to minimize forefoot pressure, while the upper material must be seamless, soft, and stretchable to reduce friction and irritation [2, 3]. The outsole should balance

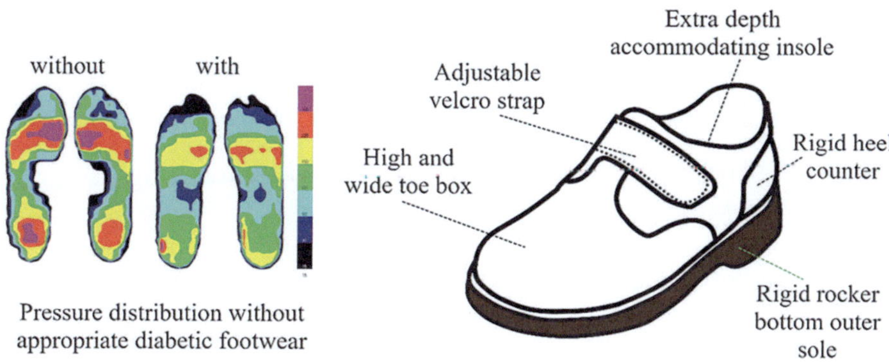


**Fig. 6.1** Plantar pressure distribution loading areas with and without appropriate diabetic footwear along with an ideal footwear for diabetic foot with important components

**Table 6.1** Footwear recommendation by risk level (IWGDF classification)

| Risk category | Footwear recommendation | Features |
|---|---|---|
| 0 | Off-the-shelf footwear | Proper fit, cushioned insole |
| 1 | Fitted footwear from trained person | Depth and soft inner lining |
| 2 | Therapeutic footwear | Custom-made insole and rocker sole |
| 3 | Medical-grade footwear | Custom-made insole, soft inner lining and insole |

rigidity for stabilization with flexibility to incorporate rocker soles, which aid in offloading pressure during gait. Adjustable closure (Velcro or laces) ensures a secure and customizable fit, and shank support enhances midfoot control. Footwear recommendations vary by risk level, as shown in Table 6.1. For low-risk patients (category 0), off-the-shelf shoes with proper fit and cushioned insoles are sufficient. Category 1 patients require fitted footwear from trained personnel, emphasizing depth and soft inner linings to prevent ulcers. Higher-risk patients (category 2) need therapeutic shoes with custom-made insole and rocker soles, while category 3 with severe deformities or prior amputations necessitate medical-grade custom shoes and insoles to mitigate recurrent injury. These guidelines prioritize pressure redistribution, structural support, and adaptability to individual foot morphology, ensuring optimal protection for diabetic patients.

Shoe modification plays a pivotal role in managing diabetic foot complications, offering targeted offloading and protection while often avoiding the need for fully custom footwear. Clinicians commonly employ evidence-based adjustments aligned with clinical guidelines and expert consensus to address specific patient needs (Table 6.2). Among the most impactful modifications is the rocker sole design, which redistribute pressure during gait; a forefoot rocker reduces stress on metatarsal heads, a double rocker offloads both forefoot and hindfoot, and a negative rocker strategically shifts weight posteriorly [4, 5]. The SACH (Solid Ankle Cushion Heel)

**Table 6.2** Shoe modification and clinical indications

| Modification | Target area | Indication | Material/technique |
|---|---|---|---|
| Rocker sole | Forefoot | Neuropathic forefoot ulcer | EVA with steel shank |
| Double rocker | Midfoot | Charcot deformity | Carbon plate and cushion layers |
| SACH heel | Heel | Ulcer or callus at heel | Rubber wedge |
| Excavation | Any | Bony prominences | Midsole foam cut-out |

modification absorbs heel strike forces and mimics plantar flexion, ideal for patients with limited ankle mobility or heel ulcers.

The common shoe modifications are commonly used in diabetic foot care. The forefoot rocker sole where the curvature (rocker) is placed just behind the metatarsal heads also referred to toe-only rocker. Its goal is to transfer load away from the forefoot. By angling the sole upward in the forefoot region, the shoe initiates the roll-over phase earlier, reducing the need for the metatarsophalangeal joints to dorsiflex during late stance of the gait cycle. This relieves pressure under the ball of the foot and toes. Forefoot rocker roles are indicated for patients with plantar forefoot ulcers, under metatarsal heads or toes, and those with limited great toe mobility (hallux limitus/rigidus) or painful metatarsophalangeal joints. They are also helpful for hammertoes or distal amputations, where reducing toe-off pressure helps to prevent ulceration at the tips of toes or at the distal end of an amputation. A properly placed forefoot rocker can reduce peak plantar pressure under forefoot and it shifts weight-bearing to the midfoot and heel effectively. Clinically one must ensure the rocker's apex or pivot point is situated proximal to ulcer or high-pressure area; often at 60–70% of the shoe length for metatarsal head offloading. Rocker angle can be 15–20° relative to floor for better offloading results. The forefoot rocker essentially substitutes for the lost motion of the toes and allow the foot to roll forward without the toes bending, thereby protecting the forefoot.

Double rocker sometimes called as a midfoot offloading rocker has two types of rockers; one under forefoot and one under heel with a relatively concave section in the middle of the outsole (Fig. 6.2). This design creates two weight-bearing points (heel and forefoot) and relieves pressure in the midfoot area by not contacting with the ground during midstance. Double rockers are especially indicated for a plantar midfoot ulcer or prominence like in Charcot foot deformity. By removing the support under the midfoot, the double rocker redistributes load to the heel and forefoot, thereby unloading a high-pressure midfoot region. Biomechanically, double rockers significantly reduce pressure at the midfoot and can reduce forefoot pressure by facilitating quicker transition to toe-off. The construction typically involves adding a thick outsole and then grinding out or designing a midfoot relief. Clinicians must ensure the two rockers are not placed too far apart and also consider the stability of the patient during gait.

The negative heel rocker modification combines a forefoot rocker with negative heel meaning the heel of the shoe sits slightly lower than the forefoot when the shoe is flat on the ground. In effect, the heel part of the sole is scooped out or lower, which causes the foot to land in a somewhat dorsiflexed position. A negative heel

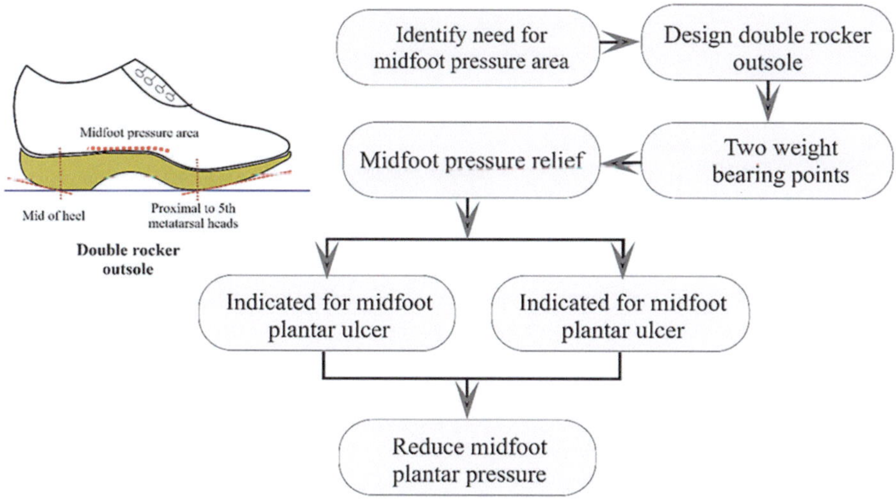


**Fig. 6.2** Double rocker shoes for the midfoot abnormal elevated plantar pressure for people with diabetic foot complications

rocker is used to offload the heel region, especially in patients with a plantar heel ulcer or a posterior calcaneal ulcer. It is also described for feet fixed in a dorsiflexed position or rigid ankle dorsiflexion contractures. By lowering the heel, weight is shifted forward toward the midfoot at stance. The negative heel reduces pressure at initial heel strike by allowing the forefoot to contact the ground sooner (essentially the opposite of a high-heeled shoe). It can also decrease pressure on the heel by distributing more pressure to the midfoot. However, it is advised to make sure; if the ankle cannot accommodate this position due to Achilles tendon tightness and the foot is normally in plantarflexion, a negative heel shoe may cause discomfort or instability. The IWGDF offload guideline does not commonly recommend negative heel shoes except in specific cases, because they can alter gait balance. In patients with a chronic heel ulcer, a negative heel rocker combined with a cushioned heel can effectively keep pressure off the calcaneus during walking. It is important to monitor for any abnormality in forefoot pressure that can alter the gait (Fig. 6.3).

Severe deformities, such as Charcot foot, may require relasting technique to reshape the midsole and outsole to accommodate structural abnormalities. Relasting refers to modifying the shape of a shoe by altering its last or by custom constructing the shoe. Relasting is used when foot shape is abnormal that even extra-depth, extra-width shoes cannot accommodate it. The primary goal is accommodation by creating a shoe that matches the foot's unique contours; relasting prevents pressure points that would occur if the foot were forced into a standard shape. A Charcot foot with a bulging medial midfoot, due to arch collapse, may require the shoe-last to be widened and reshaped in that area. Biomechanically, relasting does not add specific offloading features by itself; it ensures other modifications, such as insoles and rockers, can function without the shoe causing additional pressure.

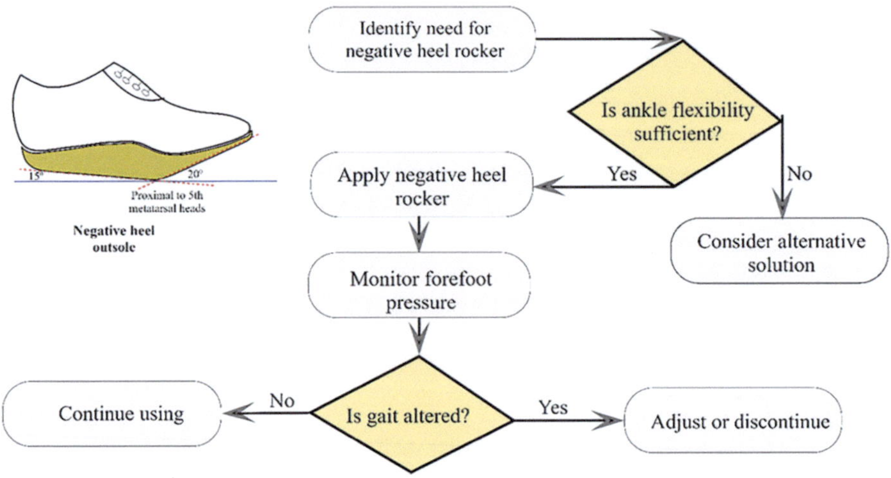


**Fig. 6.3** Negative heel modification process for people with diabetic foot complications

For localized pressure relief, the excavation technique involves carving out midsole material beneath bony prominences or high-risk areas. Upper modifications including stretching, lace-to-toe conversions, or adding balloon patches, enhance fit over deformities or post-amputation sites. Concurrently, a contralateral lift corrects limb length discrepancies caused by offloading devices like walkers, ensuring balanced gait mechanics. These tailored adjustments prioritize biomechanical optimization, ulcer prevention, and adaptability to individual foot anatomy, underscoring their value in comprehensive diabetic foot care.

A flare is an extension of the shoe's sole that widens the base on either the medial or lateral side. A medial flare extends the sole inward under the arch/heel, whereas a lateral flare extends outward. A stabilizer goes a step further, including a buildup that often encompasses part of the upper as well, creating a rigid support on one side of the shoe. Flares are indicated for patients with frontal plane instabilities: a medial flare for a pronating foot or valgus deformity and a lateral flare for an ankle that tends to invert, such as in chronic ankle sprains and varus deformity. These flares broaden the weight-bearing area and resist the tendency of the shoe to roll over to that side. Stabilizers are used for more severe instability or deformity. Both flares and stabilizers increase the shoe contact area with the ground on the side of weakness or instability, thus providing a large base of support and countering deforming forces. A medial flare, for instance, will help support a pes planovalgus by bearing some of the load that would otherwise deform the shoe inward. A lateral flare can prevent an unstable ankle from twisting by offering resistance earlier in the rollover phase of the gait cycle. Biomechanically, these modifications do not offload plantar pressure directly, but they prevent secondary shear and abnormal forces caused by instability.

## 6.4 Fitting Principles and Patient Adherence

Proper fitting of therapeutic footwear is critical for diabetic patients, particularly those with sensory neuropathy, as ill-fitting shoes are a leading cause of preventable foot ulcers. There are key checkpoints that include toe clearance, where a thumb's width (1–1.5 cm) of space should exist between the longest toe and the shoe's end to avoid compression, and measurements must be taken while the patient is standing to account for foot expansion underweight. The width must allow the foot to rest comfortably without bulging or constriction, with options for multiple widths to accommodate variations. Special attention is needed over bony prominences line bunions, ensuring the upper conforms gently without pressure. For patients using custom-made insoles, shoes must have sufficient depth (typically 5–15 mm extra depth) to avoid dorsum pressure; extra-depth styles are often ideal. The heel should be snugly cupped to prevent slippage and friction, minimizing blister risk and ulceration due to inappropriate placement during the gait. Clinicians employ tools like the Brannock device for standardized sizing and techniques such as ball-and-ring stretching to modify shoe uppers over bony prominences to provide extra room. Closure systems (laces or straps) must secure the foot without requiring toe clenching, and gait observation can detect forward sliding. After walking inspecting the foot for redness or blanching helps identify pressure points, with in-shoe pressure mapping providing objective data to ensure pressures remain below ulceration thresholds (200–250 kPa) [6]. Common fit issues arise from neuropathy-induced sensory loss, where patients may select overly tight shoes for feedback. Tight shoes causing bulging or imprints require wider sizes, stretchable uppers, or alternative styles, avoiding the break-in myth. Loose shoes leading to shear stresses may necessitate thicker socks, padding, or adjusted lacing. For mismatched foot sizes or deformities like Charcot foot require custom shoes with custom-made insole. Custom shoes should accommodate the insoles without tightness. Patients must be properly educated about shoes and insoles and should be worn incrementally (1–2 h initially) with daily foot inspections for redness, callus, discomfort, or ulcers. High-risk patients need footwear reassessment every few months due to foot structure changes. Emphasize proactive adjustments, stretching, padding, or style changes, to address evolving needs. Optimal diabetic footwear balances snug support with sufficient space to offload pressure. Fitting by foot care professional is highly advised for high-risk patients, as proper fit reduces ulcer risks, a major factor in diabetic complications. Regular follow-ups and patient education further ensure long-term foot health.

Diabetic footwear is a comprehensive approach combining design, clinical insight, and patient education. When optimized, therapeutic footwear can significantly reduce the mechanical stress that leads to ulcers, thus preserving mobility and preventing devastating outcomes. The guidelines can help clinicians to ensure that every patient with diabetes and at-risk feet has the best possible protection. It is essential to obtain properly fitting therapeutic footwear for individuals with foot conditions, diabetes, or other health issues. As technology and research advance, we can expect even more effective and personalized footwear solutions; but the core principle will remain to offload and accommodate the foot.

## References

1. Bus SA, Sacco ICN, Monteiro-Soares M, Raspovic A, Paton J, Rasmussen A, et al. Guidelines on the prevention of foot ulcers in persons with diabetes (IWGDF 2023 update). Diabetes Metab Res Rev. 2024;40(3):e3651.
2. Wang M, Li S, Teo EC, Fekete G, Gu Y. The influence of heel height on strain variation of plantar fascia during high heel shoes walking-combined musculoskeletal modeling and finite element analysis. Front Bioeng Biotechnol. 2021;9:791238.
3. Speksnijder CM, vd Munckhof RJH, Moonen SAFCM, Walenkamp GHIM. The higher the heel the higher the forefoot-pressure in ten healthy women. Foot. 2005;15(1):17–21.
4. Myers KA, Long JT, Klein JP, Wertsch JJ, Janisse D, Harris GF. Biomechanical implications of the negative heel rocker sole shoe: gait kinematics and kinetics. Gait Posture. 2006;24(3):323–30.
5. Long JT, Sirota N, Klein JP, Wertsch JJ, Janisse D, Harris GF. Biomechanics of the double rocker sole shoe: gait kinematics and kinetics. In: Conference proceedings: annual international conference of the IEEE Engineering in Medicine and Biology Society IEEE Engineering in Medicine and Biology Society Annual Conference 2004; 2004. p. 5107–10.
6. Castro-Martins P, Marques A, Pinto-Coelho L, Vaz M, Torees CJ. Plantar pressure thresholds as a strategy to prevent diabetic foot ulcers: a systematic review. Heliyon. 2024;10:e26161.

# Research Trends and Future Directions in Insole Technology, Foot Care, and AI

# 7

Muhammad Nouman and Surapong Chatpun

## 7.1 Introduction

Over the past few years, material science, biomechanical analysis, and artificial intelligence (AI) have been the engines behind the remarkable innovations in foot care and insole technology. These developments not only raise the degree of comfort and support insoles provide but also help greatly in the prevention and management of many foot-related diseases. Researchers are still looking at the link between foot mechanics and health; the possibility of creating customized insole solutions fit to the particular needs of every person is getting more appealing. These customized solutions offer choices specifically for the gait, weight distribution, and arch type of each individual, therefore revolutionizing the approach we take to foot health. Given the continuous advances in 3D printing and smart materials, insole technology seems to have huge future possibilities. This technology will be able to offer products that not only enhance performance but also help to promote overall well-being. A multidisciplinary approach must incorporate modern technologies to improve the prevention, monitoring, and treatment of diabetic foot ulcers and other podiatric conditions. Recent technological advancements, creative material applications, the function of artificial intelligence in clinical decision-making, and future foot care trends—especially with reference to diabetic foot conditions—improve quality of life. Through this analysis, we hope to show how these developments may

M. Nouman
Sirindhorn School of Prosthetics and Orthotics, Faculty of Medicine, Siriraj Hospital, Mahidol University, Bangkok, Thailand

S. Chatpun (✉)
Department of Biomedical Sciences and Biomedical Engineering, Faculty of Medicine, Prince of Songkla University, Songkhla, Thailand
e-mail: surapong.c@psu.ac.th



M. Nouman, S. Chatpun (eds.), *A Comprehensive Guide to Insole-Based Approaches for Diabetic Foot Complications*,
https://doi.org/10.1007/978-981-95-0656-9_7

significantly improve patient outcomes and quality of life. We will also discuss the concept of customized foot care solutions, which utilize data analytics and machine learning to tailor therapies to the specific needs of each patient (Fig. 7.1). These solutions not only ensure increased efficacy but also encourage a proactive approach to foot health management, as they provide support for such an approach.

## 7.2 Emerging Technologies in Foot Care and Insole Development

### 7.2.1 Smart Wearable Technology

The development of smart insoles with integrated sensors has especially helped continuous remote measurement and monitoring of plantar pressure. Essential for avoiding issues including ulceration and re-ulceration, these insoles alert consumers when plantar pressure reaches too high or higher than the threshold [1, 2]. Important markers of ulcer development and useful guides for treatment include physical elements like pressure, temperature, and humidity. Many flexible temperature sensors run on the idea that electrical resistance changes with temperature. A major advancement that will enable clinicians to more precisely evaluate ulcer situations is the inclusion of flexible temperature sensors able to digitally monitor ulcers in real time. Flexible electronics and wireless data transfer have made it simpler to create temperature sensors that detect changes in temperature while the body recovers and avoid requiring insertion into the body [3, 4]. To find out the temperature, different materials and tools are used, including conductive polymer ink, reduced graphene oxide hydrogel, and carbon-based nanotubes. All of these have been tested to see how well they work with sensor applications. Wearable technologies targeted at objectively assessing ulcer condition and controlling moisture in ulcer treatment have drawn the most attention from the research community. Using low-current digital impedance measurements, researchers have developed sterile and disposable sensors to precisely evaluate moisture content [5]. Furthermore, continuous plantar temperature monitoring using smart socks has been developed such as Siren

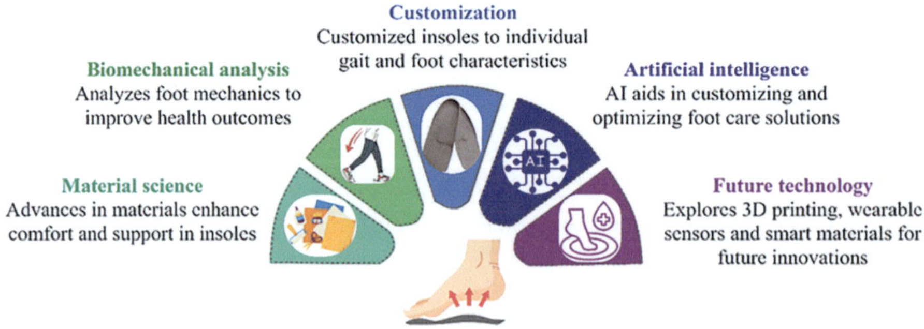


**Fig. 7.1** Revolutionizing diabetic foot health with advancement in foot care and insole technology

Diabetic Socks which can be used as an early warning system for diabetic foot ulcers [6].

Based on pressure sensing technique, pressure sensors fall into four groups: piezoresistive, capacitive, triboelectric, and piezoelectric [7]. Monitoring pressure at ulcers depends on these categories. The piezoresistive sensor was among the first kinds of sensors. Compression of its microstructures modifies its electrical resistance. The precision and dependability of the acquired data depend much on the strategic location and count of these sensors. Researchers recommend placing 15 pressure sensors around the hindfoot, midfoot, metatarsal heads, and toes to enable complete monitoring of plantar pressure [1, 8–10]. SurroSense Rx intelligent insole system (Orpyx Medical Technologies, Calgary, AB, Canada) consisted of 0.6 mm flexible pressure sensors and connected with smartwatch was implemented in high-risk diabetic patients [11]. This system provided continuous plantar pressure feedback and encouragement to offload in the daily life of patients. This study showed the better results in ulcer prevention over the long period of use, at least 6 months. The integration of diverse sensor devices into smart insoles and therapeutic footwear represents a significant advancement in foot care technology. Understanding the advantages and limitations of sensors is essential for designing effective and reliable foot care solutions. Table 7.1 shows different advantages and disadvantages of different sensor devices.

### 7.2.2 Internet of Things (IoT) Integration

The Internet of Things (IoT) is fundamentally altering our interactions with the physical world through a network of physical objects embedded with sensors, software, and network connectivity. IoT offers many opportunities for innovation, process optimization, and new business model development. The integration of IoT presents enormous potential within the healthcare sector, particularly in terms of raising capacity for portable, cost-effective, and remote patient monitoring. IoT-enabled health monitoring systems are becoming powerful tools for early-stage prevention, identification, and management of chronic diseases. These technologies support postoperative rehabilitation, enable geriatric independence promotion, and span a wide spectrum of wearable devices aimed to improve the research and development of health approaches or sports performance [13, 14]. When considering diabetic foot care for diagnosis and continuous patient physical condition monitoring, IoT devices are rather important. These systems include sophisticated sensors in smart insoles, shoes, or even straight into garments to detect significant physiological factors, including temperature, pressure, and moisture in real time. Medical professionals can track the collected data, more accurately assess health statuses, and respond fast to prevent problems by way of this continuous data collection. IoT-based systems also allow vital sign parameters to be communicated across networks of wireless sensors. In this sense, caregivers, doctors, and family members can obtain real-time patient health information. When health risks are found, this perfect information flow not only facilitates prompt and appropriate treatments but also

**Table 7.1** Advantages and disadvantages of different sensor devices [12]

| Variables | Piezoelectric sensor | Triboelectric sensor | Electromagnetic sensors |
|---|---|---|---|
| Energy conversion efficiency | High efficiency in small volume spaces | Moderate efficiency with scalability challenges | High power output but less efficient at small scales |
| Cost-effectiveness | Moderate to high, depending on material | Cost-effective | High cost to bulkier setup |
| Scalability | Limited scalability due to material fragility | High scalability potential | Limited by size and weight |
| Durability | Moderate; some materials are fragile | High durability | High durability and long-term stability |
| Applications | Best for compact, low-power devices like smart insoles | Suitable for a wide range of applications, especially where cost is a concern | Ideal for high-power applications but challenging for compact devices |
| Challenges | Material fragility and limited power<br>Fragility and limited power output | High internal electrical impedance and efficiency challenges<br>High electrical impedance and limited power output | Bulkiness and limited efficiency at small scale<br>Bulkier setup and less efficient at smaller scales |
| Key benefits | High efficiency<br>Compact design compatibility | Cost-effectiveness<br>Scalable<br>Versatile in energy capture | High power output<br>Long-term stability |

greatly helps to stop the spread of chronic disorders requiring ongoing observation. When all the elements are considered, IoT combined with footfall technology marks a major breakthrough in proactive health management, improving treatment quality and supporting patient autonomy and well-being [15, 16]. IoT technologies can help to monitor and prevent diabetic foot problems by tracking patient's physical status using sensor-equipped devices (Fig. 7.2).

### 7.2.3 AI-Driven Personalized Offloading Devices

Artificial intelligence (AI) is transforming diabetic foot ulcer prevention and management in healthcare, especially through means of AI-driven personal offloading device prescriptions. Analyzing enormous patient data, including medical history, foot shape, and walking patterns with AI, enables healthcare professionals to develop unique offloading solutions. This strategy transforms the management of diabetic foot ulcers by providing a higher level of accuracy and efficiency compared to current techniques [17]. Personalized offloading device prescriptions that are powered by AI look at and make sense of large amounts of difficult data using powerful algorithms. Using AI to analyze patients' data can help to eliminate researcher

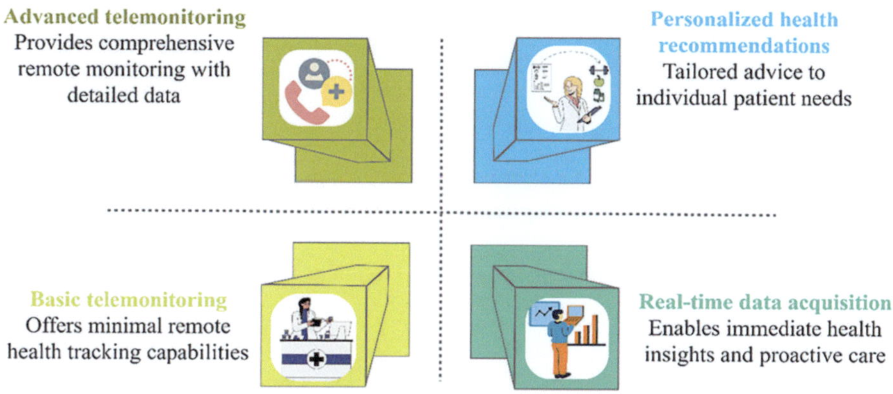


**Fig. 7.2** Impact and scenario of IoT solution in diabetic foot care

bias. Medical history, foot structure, and gait analysis are among the databases from which offloading devices, such as specialized footwear tailored to individual demands and orthotic inserts, are derived. Customizing these tools is rather important since everyone has somewhat varied unloading needs. Although national and international recommendations concur with the use of offloading devices in managing diabetic foot ulcers, their use in clinical practice is still less than ideal. For example, studies conducted in the United Kingdom revealed that hardly 5% of those with diabetic ulcers acquired a pressure-offloading device [17, 18]. Low use of these devices can be ascribed to elements including poor awareness among healthcare practitioners, insufficient training, and limited access to orthotic services. Reducing some obstacles would improve the results of therapy for diabetic foot ulcers. The improvement in accuracy and efficiency in treating diseases is one of the main benefits of offloading device prescriptions driven by artificial intelligence. By looking at human traits like foot anatomy and stride kinematics, AI systems can come up with devices that distribute pressure well and keep the plantar foot surface from being overworked. This customized strategy lowers the risk of problems and greatly raises the chances of effective ulcer healing. AI-based medications also help to increase device adherence offloading (Fig. 7.3). One main obstacle to adherence is postural instability brought on by using unloading tools, which could lead to falls during daily tasks. By analyzing biomechanical data and gait patterns, artificial intelligence algorithms can design offloading devices that reduce gait disruptions and improve stability, so addressing this problem. This, in turn, reduces the risk of falls and facilitates greater adherence to recommended offloading strategies. AI-driven solutions enable patients to have customized offloading devices without frequent in-person visits by simplifying the manufacturing and prescription writing procedures. This method guarantees patients receive fast and efficient treatment in addition to solving accessibility issues [19, 20].

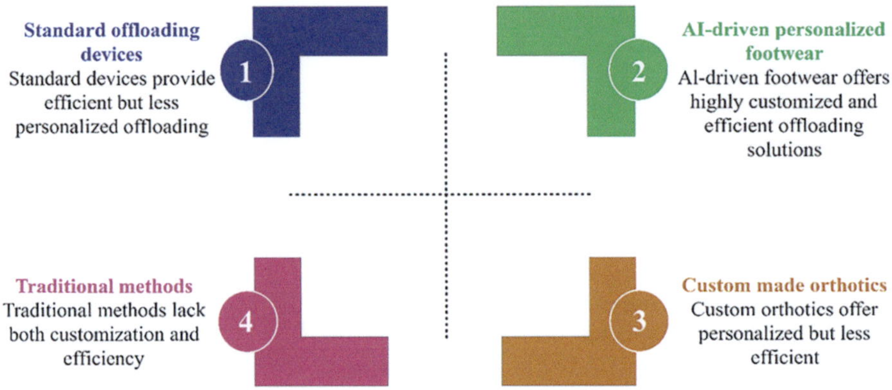


**Fig. 7.3** AI powered effectiveness in clinical decision compared to the traditional clinical practice

## 7.3 Innovations in Material Science for Insole Technology

New material technologies have greatly improved the design and functionality of diabetic foot insoles, especially when it comes to their ability to relieve pressure. Mechanical properties of insole materials affect ulcer frequency of development in diabetes patients as well as plantar pressure distribution. Though elasticity controls the regular distribution of plantar pressure and the shock absorption capacity of an insole, it is admitted as the main component in pressure release. Emphasizing the need for selecting appropriate materials for diabetic foot care, research comparing several insole materials has produced several novel suggestions for clinical usage [21–23]. With soft materials like Nora Lunalastik EVA and Poron, reducing peak plantar pressure has shown more success than with rigid alternatives [24]. For elderly patients with diabetes, these cushioned insoles help improve comfort and lower frictional stress. Research also shows that routinely softening a uniform insole can lower peak plantar pressure by as much as 30%, greatly boosting pressure redistribution and comfort [25, 26]. Moreover, the combination of soft and firm materials produces the ideal balance between comfort and structural integrity, thereby more uniformly distributing contact pressure [22, 27]. For people with diabetes, standard insole materials—plastic, rubber, and silicone—usually prove insufficient because of their nondegradable, nonabsorbable characteristics and lack of comfort. Researchers have been looking at new materials with improved mechanical properties and comfort in order to get around these limitations. Designs of single-layer, dual-layer, and multilayer insoles rely considerably on their internal structure. Different materials used in multilayered insoles give the best comfort, support, and control; especially with regard to the integration of porous patterns, structural optimization has clearly affected insole technology (Fig. 7.4). Different porous structures—such as elliptical, honeycomb, and split P Triply Periodic Minimal Surface (TPMS)—help to modify mechanical parameters like stiffness, effective modulus, and porosity, so enabling the development of quite successful tailored offloading

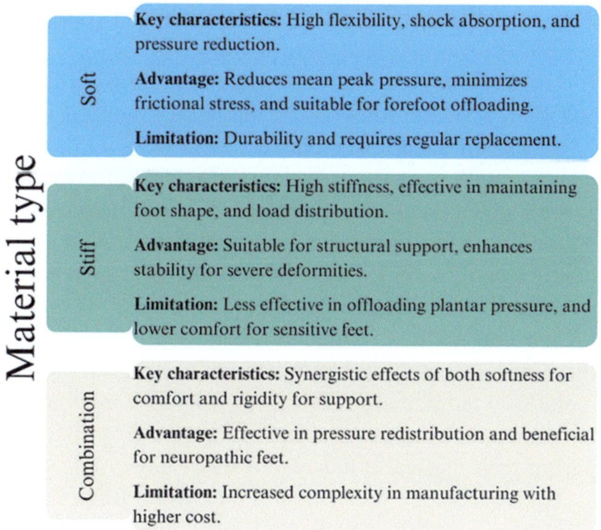


**Fig. 7.4** Material characteristics and its various functions

systems. Strong modulus and flexible geometric features of elliptical porous materials qualify them for many foot conditions. Being so incredibly rigid and load-bearing, honeycomb structures effectively reduce pressure in the forefoot and rearfoot areas. The Split P TPMS design tries to replicate medical quality foams [28]. This is an ideal substitute for diabetic foot orthoses since changing the porosity would allow different compressive strengths [29]. The developments in porous materials improve the mechanical performance of insoles and streamline the design process aiming at the foot form and load distribution. As strong 3D printing technology develops, the shift toward personalized insole designs picks speed. Using patient-specific data, 3D printing permits perfect customizing of insole geometry and material distribution, so improving fit, comfort, and the efficacy of pressure offloading. A patient-specific 3D printed insole with latticed metamaterial were fabricated to improve durability and customized stiffness over the standard of care material [30]. The infill pattern and infill density of 3D-printed insoles play an important role in pressure redistribution which can be beneficial for foot plantar pressure management for diabetic patients [31]. Moreover, useful for consistent load distribution and enhanced energy absorption are auxetic structures, defined by a negative Poisson's ratio, which increases the efficacy of diabetic foot insoles [32]. Modern materials and advanced structural designs in diabetic foot insoles should set new standards for durability, comfort, and pressure reduction. Reaching these gains totally depends on extensive testing of mechanical indicators like mechanical gradient angle, pressure time integral, pressure fluctuation index, and peak mechanical pressure. While material science advances give diabetic patients better quality of life and protection, the future of diabetic foot insoles will mostly depend on the imagination of sustainable, biodegradable, cost-effectiveness, and high-performance materials [21–23, 33, 34].

## 7.4 Clinical Trials and Evidence-Based Practice

A randomized controlled trial found that foot insoles greatly reduced peak pressure and pressure-time integrals in the hallux, lateral, and medial forefoot areas. After 12 weeks of insole use and 8 weeks following the intervention, these positive results—with a significance level of $p < 0.05$—were seen [35]. However, given the control group showed no change in their measurements during the same period, doubts about the potential long-term consequences of insoles on patient plantar loading patterns have been raised. The trial group members who used the insoles specifically reported no negative side effects. Insole modifications might incorporate several methods aimed at reducing plantar pressure in the forefoot area. These modifications include local cushioning, plastazote replacement of top coverings, metatarsal bar and arch adjustment or addition, elimination of unnecessary perforations, and arch support incorporation [36, 37]. In a 2014 Lee P.Y. et al. study comparing their clinical efficacy to a shoe-only condition, forefoot cushions drastically lowered both peak pressure and maximum force in the forefoot. With a significant level of $p < 0.001$, more specifically, the use of a plantar shield and a metatarsal dome placed 5 mm distal to the metatarsal heads resulted in reductions in peak pressure by 17% and 19%, respectively [38]. These findings suggest that, in older individuals with forefoot pain, the position of cushioning relative to the metatarsal heads may be more crucial than the specific type of cushioning itself in lowering forefoot pressures.

Customized insoles, according to study results, successfully lower plantar pressure by spreading it over several foot areas. In line with earlier studies, the redistribution of plantar pressure clearly affects the forefoot area. The study in neuropathic diabetes individuals evaluated peak plantar pressures under different walking environments. Under level walking and ramp walking without tailored insoles, the toes and forefoot showed the highest peak plantar pressure [39]. Customized insoles clearly lowered peak plantar pressure by 24.15% during level walking and by 31.77% during ramp descent. On the other hand, the heel showed a decrease of 10.2% during ramp descent; the midfoot felt more peak plantar pressure with insoles. During the first contact phase, the foot serves as a flexible body to absorb shock and then becomes a stiff body to help forward propulsion in normal gait. In diseased feet, however, aberrant gait cycles cause greater peak plantar pressures at the big toe and metatarsal heads. This is especially true of diseases such as hallux valgus. Reduced contact area during the push-off phase calls for more power to move the body. Customized insoles might assist to offset these effects by optimizing pressure distribution and increasing the contact surface, therefore improving walking comfort and lowering the risk of ulceration in diabetic patients with neuropathy [39, 40]. Patients with polyneuropathy who used insoles along with medication and wound care for 12 weeks had a significant reduction of peak pressure and pressure-time integral on hallux, medial, and lateral forefoot compared to the patients who had only medication and wound care [41]. Patient adherence to wearing insoles remains a challenge in improving the quality of life for diabetic patients.

## 7.5 Future Directions and Trends in Foot Care

Finite element analysis (FEA), recently used in foot complications evaluation, was thoroughly conducted to evaluate the distribution of plantar pressure and frictional stress in diabetic patients with neuropathy, considering pad design and material stiffness. Customized insoles (CMI) composed of various materials and their combinations underwent comprehensive FEA to assess their efficacy in lowering frictional stress and peak contact pressure. The study is significant as it emphasizes the evaluation of frictional stress across diverse CMI materials; this study is pertinent to diabetic foot care however, often overlooked in practical application [42]. In comparison to insoles constructed from firmer materials or lacking pads, the findings indicated that insoles composed of softer materials markedly reduced peak contact pressure and frictional stress at both the forefoot and hindfoot. Softer material heel pads effectively diminished the peak contact pressure of the medial and central forefoot by redistributing plantar pressure away from the rear of the foot [43]. In contrast, firmer material insoles did not demonstrate equivalent cost reductions. For CMIs composed of softer materials, such as ethylene-vinyl acetate (EVA), the peak contact pressure was significantly lower compared to thermoplastic polyurethane (TPU) and other more rigid materials. Under the first metatarsal head, a common location for ulcers in diabetes patients, softer CMIs demonstrated a significant reduction in frictional stress. Clinicians observed that osseous protrusions in the forefoot were the most common locations for the formation of ulcers and calluses. This prompted the researchers to infer, among other findings, that the forefoot endures far greater frictional stress than the rearfoot. The research associated this elevated level of frictional stress with the formation of calluses and ultimately ulcers. While prior research has indicated that frictional stresses within the shoe might result in calluses, clinical environments encounter difficulties in quantifying these pressures [44]. This study employs FEA to elucidate the impact of different CMI materials on peak plantar pressure and frictional stress, thereby assisting physicians in selecting appropriate insole materials for diabetes patients [42]. Furthermore, the FEA method enabled us to examine a real-world scenario demonstrating a balanced standing posture devoid of CMI materials in comparison. This comparative analysis highlighted the importance of material selection in effectively regulating frictional stresses and plantar pressure. The integration of AI with FEA may enhance predicted accuracy in material quality selection and the design of personalized insoles with matched with the pathological conditions. Consequently, by forecasting pressure distribution patterns and altering material combinations, AI-driven models could potentially enhance the design process further. The results indicate that the design and material selection significantly reduce the frictional stress and peak contact pressure encountered by neuropathy diabetes patients [42]. The integration of AI with FEA facilitates the development of highly tailored and resilient footbed solutions, aimed at diminishing the likelihood of foot ulcers. Several existing studies offered significant information for doctors in selecting appropriate insole materials to enhance patient outcomes by elucidating the effects of various materials on pressure and frictional stresses [42, 43, 45].

The expansion and advancement of telemedicine services allows patients to consult with podiatrists remotely, increasing accessibility and convenience. Meta-analysis showed that there was no significance difference between the telemedicine group and the face-to-face group in terms of healing rate, mortality, and healing time [46, 47]. The perceptions of 206 diabetic patients were positive with televisits, and they judged it to be useful for monitoring during the lockdown of COVID-19 pandemic [47]. This approach is particularly beneficial for routine follow-ups, managing chronic foot conditions and monitoring during the pandemic or future outbreak. Moreover, telemedicine can reduce the burden on resources and physical visits while maintaining service quality for chronic condition treatment.

## References

1. Shu L, Hua T, Wang Y, Qiao Li Q, Feng DD, Tao X. In-shoe plantar pressure measurement and analysis system based on fabric pressure sensing array. IEEE Trans Inf Technol Biomed. 2010;14(3):767–75.
2. Miller JD, Najafi B, Armstrong DG. Current standards and advances in diabetic ulcer prevention and elderly fall prevention using wearable technology. Curr Geriatr Rep. 2015;4(3):249–56.
3. Miyamoto A, Lee S, Cooray NF, Lee S, Mori M, Matsuhisa N, et al. Inflammation-free, gas-permeable, lightweight, stretchable on-skin electronics with nanomeshes. Nat Nanotechnol. 2017;12(9):907–13.
4. Huang J, Xu Z, Qiu W, Chen F, Meng Z, Hou C, et al. Stretchable and heat-resistant protein-based electronic skin for human thermoregulation. Adv Funct Mater. 2020;30(13):1910547.
5. Lu S-H, Samandari M, Li C, Li H, Song D, Zhang Y, et al. Multimodal sensing and therapeutic systems for wound healing and management: a review. Sens Actuators Rep. 2022;4:100075.
6. Reyzelman AM, Koelewyn K, Murphy M, Shen X, Yu E, Pillai R, et al. Continuous temperature-monitoring socks for home use in patients with diabetes: observational study. J Med Internet Res. 2018;20(12):e12460.
7. Naz A, Meng Y, Luo J, Khan IA, Abbas R, Yu S, et al. Cutting-edge perovskite-based flexible pressure sensors made possible by piezoelectric innovation. Materials. 2024;17(17):4196.
8. McColl D, Cartlidge B, Connolly P. Real-time monitoring of moisture levels in wound dressings in vitro: an experimental study. Int J Surg (London, England). 2007;5(5):316–22.
9. Lee HJ, Chun K-Y, Oh JH, Han C-S. Wearable triboelectric strain-insensitive pressure sensors based on hierarchical superposition patterns. ACS Sens. 2021;6(6):2411–8.
10. Pierre Claver U, Zhao G. Recent progress in flexible pressure sensors based electronic skin. Adv Eng Mater. 2021;23(5):2001187.
11. Abbott CA, Chatwin KE, Foden P, Hasan AN, Sange C, Rajbhandari SM, et al. Innovative intelligent insole system reduces diabetic foot ulcer recurrence at plantar sites: a prospective, randomised, proof-of-concept study. Lancet Digit Health. 2019;1(6):e308–e18.
12. Okoduwa SIR, Igiri BE, Tagang JI, Okoduwa UJ, Adeyi AO. Therapeutic smart-footwear approach for management of neuropathic diabetic foot ulcers: current challenges and focus for future perspective. Med Novel Technol Devices. 2024;23:100311.
13. Souza J, Escadas S, Baxevani I, Rodrigues D, Freitas A. Smart wearable systems for the remote monitoring of selected vascular disorders of the lower extremity: a systematic review. Int J Environ Res Public Health. 2022;19(22):15231.
14. Baig MM, GholamHosseini H, Moqeem AA, Mirza F, Lindén M. A systematic review of wearable patient monitoring systems – current challenges and opportunities for clinical adoption. J Med Syst. 2017;41(7):115.
15. Moncada-Sánchez LF, Salido-Ruiz RA, Espinoza-Valdez A, editors. A medical IoT-based remote monitoring system: application on diabetic foot. VIII Latin American conference on

biomedical engineering and XLII National conference on biomedical engineering. Cham: Springer; 2020.
16. Pandey R. A review on IoT based m-health systems for diabetes; 2018. p. 49.
17. Yang L, Rong GC, Wu QN. Diabetic foot ulcer: challenges and future. World J Diabetes. 2022;13(12):1014–34.
18. Jeffcoate WJ, Vileikyte L, Boyko EJ, Armstrong DG, Boulton AJM. Current challenges and opportunities in the prevention and management of diabetic foot ulcers. Diabetes Care. 2018;41(4):645–52.
19. Hassani H, Huang X, MacFeely S. Impactful digital twin in the healthcare revolution. Big Data Cognit Comput [Internet]. 2022;6(3):83.
20. Harrer S, Shah P, Antony B, Hu J. Artificial intelligence for clinical trial design. Trends Pharmacol Sci. 2019;40(8):577–91.
21. Nouman M, Chatpun S, Prachgosin T, Leelasamran W, editors. 2018 Plantar pressure distribution in non-obese, overweight and obese subjects with diabetic neuropathy while walking. 11th Biomedical Engineering International Conference (BMEiCON); 2018 21–24 Nov 2018
22. Nouman M, Chong DYR, Chatpun S. Finite element approach towards selection of appropriate materials to redistribute peak plantar pressure in diabetic foot with neuropathy: selecting appropriate materials for diabetic foot. PSU Med J. 2021;1(2):43–54.
23. Nouman M, Dissaneewate T, Leelasamran W, Chatpun S. The insole materials influence the plantar pressure distributions in diabetic foot with neuropathy during different walking activities. Gait Posture. 2019;74:154–61.
24. Shi QQ, Li PL, Yick K-L, Li N-W, Jiao J. Effects of contoured insoles with different materials on plantar pressure offloading in diabetic elderly during gait. Sci Rep. 2022;12(1):15395.
25. Chen H-Y, Chang C-K, Wang F-T, Yen C-H, Chuang H-C, Wang T-Y, et al. Effects of customized full-contact insoles crafted with polyester fabric sheets on plantar pressure and gait in hallux valgus. Bioengineering [Internet]. 2025;12(2):103.
26. Laisanitsalekul V, Srisawasdi G, Chadchavalpanichaya N, Sukthomya S. Comparison of the plantar pressure distribution between imported and local materials used for custom-made foot orthoses in patients with type 2 diabetes. J Med Health Sci. 2022;29(3):1–10.
27. Jafarzadeh E, Soheilifard R, Ehsani-Seresht A. Design optimization procedure for an orthopedic insole having a continuously variable stiffness/shape to reduce the plantar pressure in the foot of a diabetic patient. Med Eng Phys. 2021;98:44–9.
28. Jiang J, Huo Y, Peng X, Wu C, Zhu H, Lyu Y. Design of novel triply periodic minimal surface (TPMS) bone scaffold with multi-functional pores: lower stress shielding and higher mass transport capacity. Front Bioeng Biotechnol. 2024;12:1401899.
29. Claybrook F, Mohammed M, Southee D. Investigation of additive manufactured Split P TPMS elastomeric structures for diabetic foot insoles 2022.
30. Hudak YF, Li J-S, Cullum S, Strzelecki BM, Richburg C, Kaufman GE, et al. A novel workflow to fabricate a patient-specific 3D printed accommodative foot orthosis with personalized latticed metamaterial. Med Eng Phys. 2022;104:103802.
31. Chatpun S, Dissaneewate T, Kwanyuang A, Nouman M, Srewaradachpisal S, Movrin D. Infill pattern and density of 3D-printed insoles alter energy and pressure distribution in gait. Appl Sci. 2025;15(7):3916.
32. Leung MS-h, Yick K-l, Sun Y, Chow L, Ng S-p. 3D printed auxetic heel pads for patients with diabetic mellitus. Comput Biol Med. 2022;146:105582.
33. Panda B, Leite M, Biswal BB, Niu X, Garg A. Experimental and numerical modelling of mechanical properties of 3D printed honeycomb structures. Measurement. 2018;116:495–506.
34. Chen T, Tian M, Wang X, editors. A novel porous structural design of the orthotic insole for diabetic foot. 2021 International Conference on Computer, Control and Robotics (ICCCR); 2021. p. 8–10.
35. Elgohary HM, Allam I, Tolba AMN, Ali F, Alwhaibi RM, Zakaria HM, et al. Effect of foot insole on planter pressure distribution in patients with neuropathic diabetic foot ulcer: a prospective, randomized, double-blinded, controlled clinical trial. Medicina [Internet]. 2024;60(12):2066.

36. Han JT, Lee JH, Lee EJ, Lim CH, Kim WB. Comparison of plantar pressure between flat and normal feet when crossing an obstacle at different heights. J Back Musculoskelet Rehabil. 2015;28(4):629–33.
37. Xu R, Wang Z, Ma T, Ren Z, Jin H. Effect of 3D printing individualized ankle-foot orthosis on plantar biomechanics and pain in patients with plantar fasciitis: a randomized controlled trial. Med Sci Monit. 2019;25:1392–400.
38. Lee PY, Landorf KB, Bonanno DR, Menz HB. Comparison of the pressure-relieving properties of various types of forefoot pads in older people with forefoot pain. J Foot Ankle Res. 2014;7(1):18.
39. Nouman M, Leelasamran W, Chatpun S. Effectiveness of total contact orthosis for plantar pressure redistribution in neuropathic diabetic patients during different walking activities. Foot Ankle Int. 2017;38(8):901–8.
40. Guldemond NA, Leffers P, Sanders AP, Schaper NC, Nieman F, Walenkamp GHIM. Daily-life activities and in-shoe forefoot plantar pressure in patients with diabetes. Diabetes Res Clin Pract. 2007;77(2):203–9.
41. Elgohary HM, Allam I, Tolba AMN, Ali F, Alwhaibi RM, Zakaria HM, et al. Effect of foot insole on planter pressure distribution in patients with neuropathic diabetic foot ulcer: a prospective, randomized, double-blinded, controlled clinical trial. Medicina (Kaunas, Lithuania). 2024;60(12):2066.
42. Nouman M, Dissaneewate T, Chong DYR, Chatpun S. Effects of custom-made insole materials on frictional stress and contact pressure in diabetic foot with neuropathy: results from a finite element analysis. Appl Sci [Internet]. 2021;11(8):3412.
43. Nouman M, Chong DYR, Srewaradachpisal S, Chatpun S. The effect of customized insole pads on plantar pressure distribution in a diabetic foot with neuropathy: material and design study using finite element analysis approach. Appl Sci [Internet]. 2023;13(1):399.
44. Freeman DB. Corns and calluses resulting from mechanical hyperkeratosis. Am Fam Physician. 2002;65(11):2277–80.
45. Amemiya A, Noguchi H, Oe M, Takehara K, Ohashi Y, Suzuki R, et al. Shear stress-Normal stress (pressure) ratio decides forming callus in patients with diabetic neuropathy. J Diabetes Res. 2016;2016:3157123.
46. Zhuang HR, Yu HP, Gu YJ, Li LJ, Yao JL. The effect of telemedicine interventions on patients with diabetic foot ulcers: a systematic review and meta-analysis of randomized controlled trials. Adv Wound Care. 2025;14(3):133–42.
47. Yammine K, Estephan M. Telemedicine and diabetic foot ulcer outcomes. A meta-analysis of controlled trials. Foot (Edinburgh, Scotland). 2022;50:101872.

# Conclusion and Foresight

# 8

Muhammad Nouman

## 8.1 Paradigm Shift in Diabetic Foot Care

The treatment of diabetic foot complications represents a pivotal moment in modern healthcare, where clinical expertise, material science, biomechanical innovation, and technological advancement converge. This book systematically analyzes the complex difficulties surrounding diabetic foot care, highlighting the necessity of transcending traditional paradigms through multidisciplinary collaboration, biomedical engineering, and patient-centered methodologies. Three fundamental pillars emerge from the synthesis of concepts presented in previous chapters: preventive, personalized, and proactive innovation. These concepts redefine current clinical methodologies and offer a transformative framework for the future of diabetic foot care. Significant insights: a shift in perspectives on diabetic foot care complications from diabetic foot results from a combination of systemic metabolic dysregulation, localized biomechanical stressors, and individual behavioral factors; they are inherently complex. A fragmented approach to treatment, where endocrinologists, podiatrists, engineers, and rehabilitation specialists operate independently, is no longer adequate. The team-based approach is mandatory and effective, and this book illustrates the importance of integrated care techniques. Neuropathic ulcers, often caused by recurrent shear loads and elevated plantar pressure, require not just diabetes management but also biomechanical offloading and patient education regarding foot care. Multidisciplinary teams must collaborate to address the root causes of ulceration, utilizing custom-made insoles to redistribute plantar pressure and enhancing insulin regimes. Case studies from leading diabetic foot clinics

M. Nouman (✉)
Sirindhorn School of Prosthetics and Orthotics, Faculty of Medicine,
Siriraj Hospital, Mahidol University, Bangkok, Thailand
e-mail: muhammad.nou@mahidol.ac.th



M. Nouman, S. Chatpun (eds.), *A Comprehensive Guide to Insole-Based Approaches for Diabetic Foot Complications*,
https://doi.org/10.1007/978-981-95-0656-9_8

demonstrate that such partnerships can reduce ulcer recurrence rates by as much as 65% at 5 years, thereby highlighting the tangible benefits of collaborative decision-making and resource sharing [1].

## 8.2 Footwear and Insoles Beyond Ulcer Prevention

A significant advancement in diabetic foot care is the evolution of orthotic therapies from rudimentary protective devices to advanced mobility-enhancing instruments. Custom-designed insoles paired with biomechanically optimal footwear have shown to reduce peak plantar pressure by 30–50%, which correlates with a 40% decrease in ulcer occurrence [2, 3]. CAD/CAM and AI-driven design approaches provide customization tailored to dynamic gait patterns, while the materials—ethylene-vinyl acetate (EVA) and polyurethane (PU)—are intentionally layered to achieve a balance between cushioning and durability. Artificial intelligence systems that analyze pressure mapping data can now recommend insole modifications in minutes, a process that formerly needed weeks of manual iteration. In resource-constrained settings where diabetic foot problems are prevalent, these improvements enhance access to superior care and elevate clinical results. The management of diabetic foot complications represents a critical juncture in modern healthcare, where clinical expertise, material science, biomechanical innovation, and technological advancement converge. Throughout this book, we have systematically deconstructed the multifaceted challenges of diabetic foot care, emphasizing the imperative to transcend traditional paradigms through interdisciplinary collaboration, precision engineering, and patient-centered approaches. As we synthesize the insights from preceding chapters, three foundational pillars emerge; prevention, personalization, and proactive innovation. These principles not only redefine current clinical practices but also chart a transformative roadmap for the future of diabetic foot care.

## 8.3 Exercise and Rehabilitation

Tailored insoles mitigate mechanical risks; structured exercise and gait training target the physiological origins of ulcer recurrence. Chapter 5 comprehensive rehabilitation regimens demonstrate how flexibility, resistance, and balance training enhance proprioception, vascular perfusion, and musculoskeletal reliance. Patients utilizing orthotics alongside supervised exercise regimens exhibit a 35% diminished incidence of ulcer recurrence over a five-year period. Nonetheless, rehabilitation is secondary in the majority of established treatment protocols [4]. Future protocols must integrate these modalities into comprehensive treatment programs, particularly for high-risk populations such as individuals with peripheral vascular disease or Charcot foot deformities. Virtual gait training and wearable motion sensors represent developing technologies that offer innovative methods for rehabilitation, monitoring adherence, feedback, and progress, thereby closing the gap between professional recommendations and patient empowerment.

## 8.4 Future Perspectives

Anticipating the future AI-driven predictive analytics signifies a new frontier in diabetic foot care and therapy. Machine learning algorithms, trained on multimodal datasets encompassing biomechanical gait metrics, glycemic patterns, and lifestyle attributes, are prepared to enhance risk categorization through emotional analysis. Preliminary evaluations of AI-driven platforms, including those developed by prominent laboratories, demonstrated over 90% accuracy in predicting ulcer onset 6–8 weeks in advance [5, 6]. Prior to tissue degeneration, these devices offer preventative interventions such as targeted physiotherapy and dynamic insole modifications. The scalability of these tools hinges on resolving data privacy concerns and ensuring algorithmic transparency to foster clinician trust.

Using smart insoles as diagnostic tools, alongside routine treatment, represents a step toward proactive diagnosis. Situated alongside optical oxygenation monitors, thermistors, and piezoelectric sensors, these devices continuously monitor microvascular perfusion, tissue temperature, and pressure distribution. Internet of things (IoT) devices provide data transmission to alert physicians to early signs of inflammation or ischemia, enabling prompt therapies. Application areas of IoT from several laboratories have closed-loop feedback systems that autonomously adjust cushioning or rigidity of insoles in response to real-time pressure fluctuations. Despite ongoing hurdles related to durability and cost, advancements in flexible electronics, miniaturization, and energy-efficient designs are expected to facilitate the widespread adoption of these tools during the next decade.

## 8.5 Digital Twins and 3D Printing

Digital twins and additive manufacturing are emerging technologies which have been necessary and challenging to integrate. Digital twin technology is transforming insole design by creating virtual replicas of a patient's foot. By simulating pressure dynamics under different walking conditions, clinics can iteratively improve insole designs prior to physical production. This technology, in conjunction with 3D printing, enables more convenient, accurate, and faster fabrication for rapid prototyping and production of custom insoles. Furthermore, this can enhance efficiency and cost savings of insole design and fabrication. Employing digital twin-guided 3D printing to reduce material waste by 70% facilitates a reduction in manufacturing time from 3 weeks to 48 h [7]. As additive manufacturing becomes increasingly accessible, it particularly holds potential for resource-limited regions lacking traditional orthotic fabrication systems. Despite technological advancements, disparities in diabetic foot care persist. Low- and middle-income nations comprise over 80% of amputations; access to specialists and contemporary orthotic devices remains limited in these regions. Leveraging technological advancements and fostering collaborations among healthcare experts can facilitate the creation of a more inclusive diabetic foot care strategy that addresses the specific requirements of marginalized populations.

## 8.6 Bridging Knowledge Gaps

Despite a deficiency in understanding biomechanical principles or proficiency with digital tools, clinicians continue to be the cornerstone of diabetic foot care. Medical curricula must evolve to include modules on wearable technologies, design thinking, orthotic design, and interdisciplinary care coordination. Tools like augmented reality can facilitate the visualization of plantar pressure redistribution, while simulation-based training enhances practical skills. Alongside patient education programs such as smartphone applications that instruct self-monitoring techniques can empower individuals to engage actively in their treatment.

Continued longitudinal studies are needed to validate AI, wearable, and 3D printing technologies in diverse diabetic populations. Diabetic foot care is no longer a reactive practice; it is a proactive frontier of innovation, equity, and empowerment. Through clinical integration, emerging technology, and community-focused delivery models, these can shift the narrative of diabetic foot management from one of chronic risk to one of restored function and dignity.

## References


1. Armstrong DG, Tan T-W, Boulton AJM, Bus SA. Diabetic foot ulcers: a review. JAMA. 2023;330(1):62–75.
2. Ahmed S, Barwick A, Butterworth P, Nancarrow S. Footwear and insole design features that reduce neuropathic plantar forefoot ulcer risk in people with diabetes: a systematic literature review. J Foot Ankle Res. 2020;13(1):30.
3. Hellstrand Tang U, Zügner R, Lisovskaja V, Karlsson J, Hagberg K, Tranberg R. Comparison of plantar pressure in three types of insole given to patients with diabetes at risk of developing foot ulcers – a two-year, randomized trial. J Clin Transl Endocrinol. 2014;1(4):121–32.
4. Bęcławska S, Błażkiewicz M, Czyżewski P, Rutkowski T, Wąsik J. Home-based lower limb exercises for individuals with diabetes: a scoping review. Appl Sci. 2025;15(8):4552.
5. Hasan MH, Nil S, Sourov MN, Nishi J, Shidujaman M, Habib M. AI-driven smart device for non-invasive detection of peptic ulcers for sustainable healthcare; 2025. p. 1386–91.
6. Cassidy B, Hoon Yap M, Pappachan JM, Ahmad N, Haycocks S, O'Shea C, et al. Artificial intelligence for automated detection of diabetic foot ulcers: A real-world proof-of-concept clinical evaluation. Diabetes Res Clin Pract. 2023;205:110951.
7. Kantaros A, Piromalis D, Tsaramirsis G, Papageorgas P, Tamimi H. 3D printing and implementation of digital twins: current trends and limitations. Appl Syst Innov. 2022;5(1):1–13.

MIX
Papier aus verantwortungsvollen Quellen
Paper from responsible sources
FSC® C105338

If you have any concerns about our products,
you can contact us on
**ProductSafety@springernature.com**

In case Publisher is established outside the EU,
the EU authorized representative is:
**Springer Nature Customer Service Center GmbH**
**Europaplatz 3, 69115 Heidelberg, Germany**

Printed by Libri Plureos GmbH
in Hamburg, Germany